Oral Self Care
Strategies for Preventive Dentistry

Hygienist's Edition

Philip Weinstein, Ph.D.
Peter Milgrom, D.D.S.
with
Lisa J. Heaton, Ph.D.

Library of Congress Cataloging in Publication Data

Main entry under title:

Oral Self-Care

Bibliography:

ISBN: 0-9779618-2-6

Published by:

Dental Behavioral Resources
Seattle, Washington
http://www.dentalbehavioralresources.com

10 9 8 7 6 5 4 3 2 1

Printed in the United States of America

Contributors

Philip Weinstein, Ph.D.
Professor, Department of Dental Public Health Sciences
University of Washington School of Dentistry
Seattle, Washington, USA

Peter Milgrom, D.D.S.
Professor, Department of Dental Public Health Sciences
University of Washington School of Dentistry
Seattle, Washington, USA

Lisa J. Heaton, Ph.D.
Senior Fellow, Department of Dental Public Health Sciences
University of Washington School of Dentistry
Seattle, Washington, USA

Tarja Kaakko, D.D.S.
Assistant Professor, Department of Pediatric Dentistry
University of Washington School of Dentistry
Seattle, Washington, USA

Contents

Acknowledgments

Foremost we would like to express our sincere appreciation to our patients, without whose assistance this book could not be written.

We are indebted to our clinic staff—assistants, dental hygienists, and dentists, who have encouraged our ideas and spurred us on to innovate. We would in particular like to recognize the hygienists Marilynn Rothen, and Gail Heacox and assistants Sharon Lawrence and Shelly Petersons of the Dental Fears Research Clinic at the University of Washington who are willing to try our ideas and give us feedback.

We wish to salute our new collaborator, Lisa Heaton, who has joined the authors of this book and has made many useful and insightful additions to this work. Although we maintain overall responsibility for the contents of this text, we have specifically acknowledged Lisa's primary authorship of several chapters so that her talents and contributions will be recognized.

We thank Doug Ramsay, our department chair and friend, for the opportunity to teach a seminar for graduate students in the specialty training programs in Orthodontics and Pediatric Dentistry that led to the chapter in this new edition.

We are grateful to Reinhard "Ron" Hahn for applying his expertise in monograph layout, typological design and camera-ready copy production to this work. With his numerous skills and talents, he transformed our words and images into a polished final product.

We also thank Mary Martin for her editing expertise and valuable suggestions for improving this text. Her endless energy and keen eye helped pull this work together into a cohesive whole.

Two of our most important collaborators have retired since the publication of the 3rd edition of *Oral Self Care: Strategies for Preventive Dentistry*. We particularly acknowledge Agnes Spadafora who for years guided us with her wit and clinical wisdom. We wish her well. Tracy Getz served as coauthor of the earlier additions and was often the engine that got projects moving. He is in active retirement and we hear from him often. We miss his contributions and clinical experience.

Philip Weinstein, Ph.D.

Peter Milgrom, D.D.S.

Seattle, Washington, August 2006

Oral Self Care :
Strategies for Preventive Dentistry

Hygienist's Edition

Philip Weinstein and Peter Milgrom with Lisa J. Heaton

"Lots of folks confuse bad management with destiny.

E. Hubbard"

Introduction to the Fourth Edition

We are pleased to present the fourth edition of *Oral Self Care: Strategies for Preventive Dentistry*. This edition has been planned for quite a while, as there is much new knowledge we desired to incorporate into this book in the fifteen years since the last edition. The third edition became a classic, used particularly in dental hygiene and assisting programs throughout the United States and in translation in a number of other countries. As we lectured throughout the world, fellow professors from a myriad of settings adopted the textbook for their classes and practitioners from varied lands have incorporated our tips and ideas into practice.

Taking the prevention of dental disease seriously can be an exercise in frustration. Unfortunately patients do not often follow through on our treatment plans or respond to our recommendations for home care. The traditional "tell them what to do" health education approach has many limitations. This text was written to provide students and practitioners with an arsenal of new ideas to enhance their success in this difficult area.

Behavior change technology is an important part of all the editions of this text. While this technology remains essentially the same, there have been other psychological studies relevant to students and practitioners attempting to prevent dental disease. The understanding of patient readiness to act and new and proven motivational approaches are now available to dental personnel. Such approaches fit well with the use of behavioral change technology. While in its infancy, these approaches have been research tested and clinically applied in both private dental practice and public health settings.

The distinction in this text between short term and long- term goals is an important one. While acute episodes occur, dental diseases are chronic disorders. Short term fixes, e.g., fillings and extractions, are not able to control dental diseases. At times, perhaps because of the surgical orientation of many dental providers, patients believe that dental treatment itself is capable of controlling dental disease (which it is not).

Dental patients returning to see assistants, hygienists, and dentists is the sine qua non of successful prevention. It is impossible to control dental disease without repeated visits and continuity of care. Given that patients accept that returning to see dental personnel over time is a normative behavior that is expected in our society, we have the opportunity to break up the problem into manageable pieces, with short-term goals and behavioral methodologies. Moreover, we do not have to adhere to a recall appointment every six moons. Patient recall intervals can reflect patient dental needs and can compensate for temporary deficiencies in oral self-care.

There have been a number of innovations in the chemotherapeutic management of dental disease since the last edition. These approaches are discussed in the "Therapeutic Alternatives" chapter. These advances aid the clinician in preventing and controlling oral disease while behavioral changes are taking hold. They also allow for the ups and downs of the collaboration between patients and clinicians and help avoid staff burnout. The chapter addressing "Working with Orthodontic Patients" is an important new application of these concepts.

There have been other changes in the text from the previous edition. The chapter entitled, "Communicating With Your Patients" focuses on communication skills and is followed by a chapter that uses these skills to assess and motivate patients. Our recent work in Motivational Interviewing is highlighted.

While smoking is frowned upon by our society, a substantial minority of the population smokes. Given that tobacco causes oral cancers and that dental personnel are primary care providers, the "Smoking Cessation" chapter was written to provide up-to-date smoking cessation strategies. Special populations are addressed again in this edition with completely revised chapters on oral self care for children (and teens) and patients with special needs and the elderly. This edition also attempts to further the student and practitioners' awareness and skill in addressing individual differences. Discussions of mental health issues are included in the text.

In all, this text provides the reader with a state-of-the-art clinical application of behavioral sciences to the problem of preventing and controlling dental disease. Just as reading a book or watching a video on fly-fishing will not put fish in your creel, simply reading this book is not enough. We believe you can best master our approach and techniques by trying them out. We suggest you identify a real problem you want to work on as you read this book. Let us know how it goes.

Part I:

DEFINING THE PROBLEM

"

I want to change things.
I want to see them happen.
I don't want to just talk about them.

J. K. Galbraith

"

Chapter 1

Why Most Plaque Programs Do Not Work

Nature and Magnitude of the Problem in Prevention

Scientific findings in the 1960s and early 1970s indicated that dental caries and periodontal diseases are largely preventable. Dentists, dental hygienists, and assistants responded by instituting plaque control programs. Initial studies from private practice reported rapid improvement in oral hygiene following home-care instruction. However, by the mid 1970s enthusiasm faded as these efforts failed to produce long-term changes in patient hygiene. Studies often revealed regression back to initial levels of plaque and calculus (Lindhe and Koch, 1964). At best, this research has shown that without intermittent professional supervision, most patients who initially follow new home-care instruction do not maintain the behavior.

Success with one out of two patients in teaching regular brushing and/or flossing is considered a good result. In a university based study of periodontal patients who rinsed with chlorhexidine, we found that only one-half used the rinse fully as instructed. This closely matches the 50-percent rate of adherence reported for long-term medical regimens. Results are often less than 50 percent. For example, in a review article, Wilson (1998) reported a noncompliance rate of 11 to 45 percent in university-based periodontal disease maintenance programs and a compliance rate of one in three or less in private practice settings. Nonetheless, our success with individual patients in clinical practice encourages us to try to find the principles underlying successful behavior change so we can apply them to more patients.

Starting a habit change is difficult, but maintaining long-term gains has proved even more difficult. Research indicates that two-thirds of patients who drop out of preventive programs do so within 90 days. Not only is there a decline in participation in preventive programs over time, but when professional attention has ended, effects of the programs are not maintained. This might explain why in our studies of patients in private practices, most patients on three- and six-month recall had plaque levels no different at recall from their levels before treatment and oral hygiene instruction (Weinstein and Milgrom, 1988).

On the other hand, some evidence indicates that people are capable of altering their self-care behaviors even without professional assistance. Shachter (1982) reported that successful long-term changes in behavior for smoking, obesity, and drug use, initiated by motivated individuals alone, are relatively common. Over repeated attempts, large numbers of individuals have been successful in changing behavior by themselves. Although a single recommendation or specific attempt at teaching a patient a cleaning skill may not be completely successful, the probability of success from a series of well-timed professional efforts is substantially greater, especially after rapport and trust are established.

Compliance and Self-Care

Historically, preventive activities have been viewed from a compliance perspective (Sackett and Snow, 1979). The term *compliance* defines a provider-oriented rather than a patient-oriented frame of reference. The model of the doctor-patient relationship is authoritarian; the doctor gives instructions to the patient, who is expected to comply. The ideal portrayed is that of a passive, submissive patient. The patient's current self-care behaviors are not usually investigated.

The compliance model warrants rethinking, since treatment of chronic dental diseases, including caries and forms of periodontal disease, requires a high proportion of self-care relative to professional care. Self-care has been and continues to be a substantial factor in the success or failure of health care. Studies in a variety of settings indicate that many self-care practices are nearly universal, and without them any health-care system would be ineffective. However, little research has been conducted in understanding self-care activities and how they interrelate with and influence the acquisition of new care behaviors.

Activities of daily living require self-care. Bathing and toothbrushing are examples often provided to describe habitual behavior that is self-initiated, self-maintained, and self-monitored. In all, socialization of the child, together with some supplementary formal health education, "contributes a myriad of living ... behaviors which are taken for granted as a sort of base line of responsible human activities" (Levin, 1977, p. 12).

Brushing one's teeth is an activity of daily living and need not be viewed strictly in terms of compliance or noncompliance. Studies indicate that oral hygiene is practiced regularly in all cultures. For example, Smith and Striffier (1963) reported that 86 percent of their sample of American males and 98 percent of females brushed at least once per day. Similarly, Sheiham (1970) reported that 99.5 percent of adult British females and 90 percent of British males brushed daily. Differences between social classes were not great. Moreover, there was evidence that the majority of the British population brushed two or more times a day.

Blinkhorn (1978) found toothbrushing to be a part of the primary socialization process for the majority of British children; 54 percent began brushing before age 2, and mothers played the most important role in establishing the brushing habit. However, Blinkhorn was dismayed to find that only 20 percent of the total sample of mothers had received any professional advice on how to look after their children's teeth. He concluded that dental health professionals "have failed to assist the mothers who are interested in caring for their children's teeth" (p. 224). This conclusion placed primary responsibility on the dental health professional. Other conclusions are possible: that cultural norms for oral self-care behaviors exist and that individuals adopt normative patterns of self-directed health regimens.

The concept of dentist- or preventative therapist-imposed care activities versus self-initiated care behaviors in the context of cultural or subgroup norms raises interesting questions about the role of the professional. We believe that helping to refine *already existing* self-care patterns leads to higher long-term rates of oral hygiene activities than attempting to get patients to comply with prescribed regimens. Overall, the concept of compliance has built-in inadequacies, especially in attempts to establish long-term preventive behaviors. Approaching the problem by examining the patient's existing self-care habits and his or her unique difficulties in altering existing behaviors is, we believe, more useful.

Why do we have such difficulty improving a patient's oral care when the majority of individuals perform it on a regular basis? We believe there are several problems that function to minimize the effectiveness of programs designed to improve a patient's home care. We will discuss each in turn and suggest ways to mitigate its effect.

Problem 1.
Plaque-control programs begin too early.

In most practices, patients are routinely scheduled into a plaque-control program *prior* to dental treatment, often at the initial diagnostic appointment! Though well meaning and efficient, this approach results in difficulties for plaque control programs.

To influence patient thinking and actions, dental practitioners must establish rapport and trust and be aware of the individual's perceived dental needs. Reasonable goals must also be set. When we begin plaque-control programs before we learn about the individual, there is no way to personalize our preventive message; moreover, patients often need repeated visits for dental care to learn about their problems and focus attention on areas that are high priority for attention at home. *Oral hygiene instruction during, and especially after, restorative and periodontal care can be very effective.*

Problem 2.
Plaque control often begins without patient ownership or readiness.

This problem is usually closely associated with Problem 1. Dentists, dental hygienists, and assistants who function as preventive therapists usually do not determine whether or not *the patient* feels he or she has (owns) a problem and perceives there is a deficit worth working on at this time. Too often it is the dentist or therapist who really owns the problem; that is, it is he or she, not the patient, who desires the change.

Though there is little work in this important area, the research of Starfield *et al.* (1981) supports this position. These investigators found that practitioner-patient agreement about problems was associated with greater patient expectation for involvement and better health outcomes than when only the practitioner believed a problem existed.

Not everyone is ready to change self-care habits. Some are never ready. Social pressure from the dental hygienist may result in superficial acquiescence, but attempts to try out the new self-care behavior may be minimal. The self-care approach addresses the issue of responsibility for patient behavior by helping the patient identify his or her need to change oral self-care practices.

Paradoxically, the professional's responsibility is greater with the compliance approach. There is no need to determine patient need or ownership of the problem, because the practitioner does all the work. On the other hand, with the self-care approach the practitioner attempts to determine patient perceptions of need and responsibility. Once the patient "owns" or identifies the problem and the benefits associated with solving the problem, it is appropriate for the practitioner to take some responsibility in assisting the patient to change both skill and habit

Initially, before the patient perceives that a problem worth acting upon exists, information from the professional will be "hit or miss;" that is, information that is not targeted toward patient concerns is unlikely to hit its mark. At this point, it is important for the professional to ask good, engaging, open-ended questions and then to listen.

Such questioning uncovers patient concerns and desires. For example, "Tell me about your teeth and what you want from them?" or, "What would you like if we could give you 'a dental make-over'?"

If the patient does not identify a need after questioning and listening, and thereby shows he does not desire to change, there is little a practitioner can do to help at that time. Nonetheless, contact with the patient over several years may yield a period when even the patient stuck in deepest denial concerning dental health may become interested. All along, the therapist should identify patient stage of readiness and provide appropriate responses. We believe a major reason for the high failure rate of prevention and the "burnout" of therapists is lack of recognition of differences among patients and their stages of readiness.

Problem 3.
Lack of a personal approach to plaque control efforts.

Communication is critical. Dentist, hygienists, and assistants must take considerable care in introducing plaque-control programs. Gold (1974) notes that although many dentists tell their patients about plaque control, most are unaware that how they are relating this information is more important than *what* they are relating. Davis (1968) found that "patterns of communication which deviate from the normative doctor-patient relationship will be associated with failure" (p. 287). Such patterns include terse interaction and situations where the clinician is perceived as formal, rejecting, or controlling, or where he or she disagrees overtly with the patient, or talks to the patient at length and does not provide an opportunity for feedback. While these studies are a generation old, unfortunately they are still relevant.

For example, many patients believe they are already doing an acceptable job of cleaning. The patient may feel slighted or coerced by the dental professional's comments and suggestions, which may intimate he or she is "incompetent" in oral self-care. Dental professionals must be careful in introducing plaque control; merely to raise the topic may cause patients to infer that their care habits are being criticized.

Dental educators usually stress the importance of "cleaning up the patient's mouth" *prior* to definitive dental treatment. Again, this approach may cause difficulties for plaque-control programs. To influence patient thinking and actions, dental practitioners must be aware of the individual's dental needs and help establish short- and long-term goals. When a dentist begins a plaque-control program before learning about the individual, there is no way to personalize the preventive message. Consequently, the motivational appeal to the patient is often "canned," not personalized. The act of motivating a patient involves asking questions, listening (which shows concern), and then providing information. Our own interest and commitment to prevention are important factors. If we are not enthusiastic and do not believe in the efficacy of preventive activities, we will communicate this attitude to the patient.

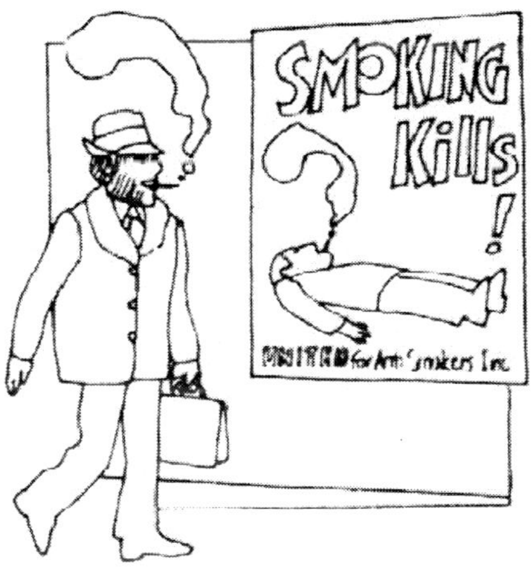

Similarly, concern about the welfare of the patient is very important. Patients usually judge concern by the amount of time the therapist spends listening and discussing their health and their problems. Information provided need not be technical, but it must be relevant. Patients need to understand why the information is important and how it relates to them personally. Directing the patient to examine his or her own mouth and helping the patient observe diseased tissue, plaque remaining after cleaning, etc., is very useful.

However, the research literature firmly indicates that merely giving information, the "why" of prevention, does not lead to altered behavior. As Evans (1978) notes, certain myths permeate our health education efforts. One myth is that if sufficient information is communicated and the patient understands the etiology of the disease and the effectiveness of preventive health practice, his or her behavior will change. However, as an illustration of the fallacy in this belief, consider that by the time they reach seventh grade almost all children have heard that smoking is dangerous to their health, yet about 20 percent of them are already smoking. Old myths die hard, and many practitioners continue to believe that simply providing information to the patient will lead to improvements in self care.

Actually, as we have already said, providing information is often of secondary concern in motivating patients. Asking questions and listening is primary. Unfortunately, dental professionals tend to provide much too much information. We seem to think that a patient needs to be taught oral microbiology. We talk too much. Moreover, to maximize the chances of motivating patients to think and act in different ways, the message must be personalized, not "canned." Questioning and listening skills are especially important. Audiovisual materials are helpful in providing information, but they are no substitute for interest and concern for the individual. For prevention to work, communication must be two-way. Patient airtime is essential and must be encouraged.

Problem 4.
Our assumptions about the reasons for patient nonperformance of plaque control are often mistaken.

When we find a patient who is not flossing at all, for example, we may hear the therapist state that the patient either does not know how to floss or does not know how important flossing is; otherwise, he or she obviously would be flossing. Such statements talk about solutions, not problems. Instruction in health care is a solution for a lack of information. Frequently, however, lack of information is not the problem. We have found that when there is a gap between a patient's desired performance and his or her actual performance (which we call a *performance discrepancy*), It is usually a function of a lack of skills in establishing and maintaining a long-term habit. Though a patient may be motivated to think differently and try out a new home-care behavior, health professionals both in medicine and dentistry have paid scant attention to helping the patient manage his or her behavior. Have you been motivated enough to try a new diet or exercise program? Have you been in a physical therapy program? Did you ever get any help in making it stick? Probably not. Dental patients also face these problems.

Problem 5.
Old habits are automatic.

This is a very common problem, and one that is difficult to overcome. Most of us have been brushing our teeth since early childhood, and it is something we perform without thinking. We daydream about what we will do next, what we should have done at the office today, etc., as we perform a skill that in fact calls for concentration and attention.

Problem 6.
We assume that the patient has adequate skills to clean adequately.

Careful assessment of existing patient self-care practice may be very important. Though plaque-control instruction often focuses on skill training, dentists, hygienists, and assistants often do not systematically evaluate patient skills *prior* to instruction. Though time-consuming, such effort is invaluable in tailoring instruction to patient needs and gaining greater patient acceptance.

Knowledge of how the patient cleans can only come from observation. It is our experience that when asked to demonstrate skills, patients attempt to perform optimally. In such situations, there is social pressure to spend more time cleaning and to clean more thoroughly. As patients attempt to avoid embarrassment, awkward, unfamiliar manipulations of instruments may be evident.

Problem 7.
We try to teach too much, too quickly.

It is common to teach the patient how to clean all of his or her teeth in one sitting. It is, after all, a small area and a task that takes a skilled person only a few minutes to perform. However, given the amount of dental disease in this country, it apparently is a task which must be more difficult than it first appears. As we have already discussed, there are several reasons why it is a difficult task. For the person with "fair" or "poor" hygiene, we are much more successful in teaching cleaning skills and follow-through at home when we break the task into smaller steps. Ideally, we like to concentrate on only one instrument until it is fully mastered, starting with the brush and gradually introducing other necessary tools. Second, we try to pair our hygiene instruction with the actual work being performed. For example, after we provide subgingival curettage and root planing in a quadrant, we demonstrate the specific techniques on how to keep up the newly cleaned area. Until the patient shows mastery at that skill, we do not move on to other areas of the mouth or to more complex cleaning procedures. Similarly, we never ask a patient to clean posterior teeth until the more visible, anterior ones are successfully cleaned.

Problem 8.
Plaque-control programs lack adequate follow up.

Dental researchers investigating the efficacy of plaque-control programs have reported that changes in oral-health habits seldom last more than six months. Long-term change of oral-hygiene patterns is difficult, involving skills in self-control and restructuring habit patterns. We have developed techniques that facilitate maintenance of long-term habits. Follow-up calls and visits after teaching how to clean a new area are essential for most patients. Teaching patients to accept occasional lapses so they will not return (relapse) to old, ineffective habit patterns is another important area.

Problem 9.
Plaque control is not financially rewarding.

Besides the frustration of trying to promote preventive activities to resistant patients, dental practitioners must face the present reality that preventive activities do not generate much income. Nonetheless, data generated by the American Dental Association show that upwards of one-half of the hours of a typical practice are now devoted to preventive-diagnostic services. In a day when dentists can hire and delegate to well-trained paraprofessionals, fees paid by the patient can compensate the preventive therapist for time spent. New types of insurance programs, especially capitation programs, can be expected to foster this trend. However, in the past, practitioners faced with a probability of little patient benefit and the poor financial reward tended to minimize preventive activities.

In short, patients get what they pay for. We believe that financial incentives for the dental provider are important and must be built into plaque-control programs. In our own clinical practice, we charge patients for time spent in preventive activities. The faster they progress in their preventive activities (and require fewer office visits), the lower the cost. More useful and practical, however, has been more frequent recall after a series of restorative and/or periodontal treatments. Patients readily accept and pay for the need to polish a filling or check periodontal health. This gives us a chance to review and enhance preventive skills

Problem 10.
Plaque control programs are often not offered to those who need it most.

Our clinical research, which involved tape recording many private practice preventive sessions, leads to the conclusion that more plaque control instruction is offered to healthy than diseased patients. The patient with more extensive disease is often seen as uninterested or unwilling. On the contrary, our experience is that this patient is extremely desirous of improved health but is rarely offered plaque control in a step-by-step approach that will succeed. Because a patient has poor oral health and is now seeking care, he or she is a very important and often receptive audience.

Problem 11.
Personnel turnover in the practice defeats education efforts.

Changes in personnel and the dental hygienist shortage are problems. However, we have found that failure by the dentist to allow personnel to individualize care and spend more time with sicker patients feeds the turnover problem. Skilled hygienists and assistants are in great demand today, and many simply refuse to work in practices where the dentist will not allow personnel to spend more time and effort with patients who need it. Bravo!

In conclusion, when dental professionals manage their preventive practices based on a compliance model, no more than half the patients respond. Self-care formulations appear to present real advantages and present possibilities for enhancing success. Most important, although the compliance approach ignores the influence of present self-care activities, the self-care approach identifies and fosters patient readiness and builds upon the patient's current behaviors. We can help people make their existing habits more efficient and effective without necessarily adding minutes to home-care regimens, thereby minimizing the possibility of patient rejection. This self-care model also recognizes the difficulty of transferring skills from the office to the home and attempts to minimize interference from existing, nonfunctional self-care behaviors.

"

When people talk, listen completely.
Most people never listen.

E. Hemingway

The greatest compliment that was ever paid me was
when someone asked me what I thought, and
attended to my answer.

H. D. Thoreau

"

Chapter 2

Communicating with Your Patients

Health Literacy – What do people know?

Think back to the last time you brought your car to the mechanic or sat down to discuss finances with an accountant. You may have found that at times, this person used terms that you were not familiar with, such as "crank shaft pulley" or "portfolio diversification." If you felt comfortable enough with the person to ask what those terms meant, you could get the information you needed. If you did not feel comfortable, however, you may have simply nodded and made a note to yourself to look up that information later or ask someone you trust.

Similarly, many of the terms and concepts we use in dentistry can sound foreign to patients. A primary goal of dental professionals, then, is to educate patients about dental care while keeping in mind the levels of knowledge and understanding they have about oral health. We refer to this knowledge as *oral health literacy*, and it must be taken into account for each individual patient we treat.

Oral health literacy has been the recent focus of a national initiative. Its purpose is to assess how well individuals are able to understand information (particularly written materials) related to oral health. The initiative grew out of previous research that suggests a significant percentage of adults in the United States are not able to read and/or understand written health information materials. It is reasonable to expect that many individuals have difficulty reading and/or understanding information related to oral health as well. Dental patients obtain information about oral health and dental care from a variety of sources, and they bring this information to the dental office. We will now turn to the types of questions, information (and misinformation) that patients may present to you in your practice.

How do we assess what our patients know?

Overall, the questions patients ask can give you a good idea of their levels of health literacy. People use many sources to gain information about health. The particular sources your patients use will be communicated in their questions. Here are the primary sources patients use:

Personal sources, such as friends, family members, and acquaintances. Patients will report things they've been told by people around them who they trust. Be careful not to discredit these sources, because this will immediately put patients on the defensive. Some things NOT to say:

- "Well, your friend must have picked a really bad dentist, if she had that happen."
- "It sounds like your sister may have overreacted to what the hygienist said."
- "I think your father was just trying to scare you when he said you were going to lose all your teeth."

Media Sources, such as popular television programs, web sites, and magazines (but not dentistry journals or oral health web sites). Many patients receive the majority of their health information through popular media that give the impression of impartial, objective information. Although some popular media sources provide good information, some gain people's attention by using scare tactics. For example, a news program may run a story about the dangers of mercury in amalgam fillings. A clinician who discredits the report may make patients feel foolish by making remarks such as:

- "That magazine runs garbage like that just to sell more subscriptions."
- "Well, you can't believe anything you see on that channel."

- "That story was so one-sided it was ridiculous."

Professional sources, such as oral health journals and websites (American Dental Association, American Medical Association, etc.) may prompt questions from some patients. It is important to reinforce patients for seeking out good information. For example, you can say something like, "The ADA website is a great resource. Did you have any more questions about the information you found there?" Conversely, you should NOT say:

- "Wow! How did YOU get a hold of this information?"
- "Did someone help you with this?"
- "I'll bet that this information was kind of over your head. Let me help you understand it."

References for Patients

With regard to professional sources, there are several online sources that you may recommend to patients in addition to any materials you may have in your office:

American Dental Association, Consumer Information

`http://www.ada.org/public/index.asp`

Dental Health (MedLine Plus)

`http://www.nlm.nih.gov/medlineplus/dentalhealth.html`

Basic Dental Care (WebMD)

`http://www.webmd.com/hw/dental/hw144416.asp`

Tooth Disorders (MedLine Plus)

`http://www.nlm.nih.gov/medlineplus/toothdisorders.html`

Dental Caries/Tooth Decay (WebMD)

`http://www.webmd.com/hw/dental/hw172498.asp`

Cosmetic Dentistry (MedLine Plus)

`http://www.nlm.nih.gov/medlineplus/cosmeticdentistry.html`

Dentures (MedLine Plus)

`http://www.nlm.nih.gov/medlineplus/dentures.html`

Of course, not all resources on the Internet are reputable, and patients may find inaccurate information as they search the Web. It can sometimes be difficult to tell a reputable web site from one with inaccurate information. Encourage your patients to seek out sites from national organizations, such as the American Dental Association (ADA), National Institutes of Health (NIH), and American Medical Association (AMA), or from University-based web sites. These sites include pages written for consumers, avoiding overly technical terms. In addition, reputable sites usually cite their sources, such as peer-reviewed journals. Many private dental practices have web sites that include dental information such as "teeth whitening" and "sedation dentistry." However, patients should be cautious in basing decisions on privately owned web sites, because the focus of some of these sites may be on selling a product or a treatment rather than on providing objective information.

Patients may have incorrect assumptions or information about oral health. When we are presented with questions that seem rather "common sense" to dental professionals, it is most important *not* to make patients feel as though they have asked "a silly question." If a patient asks a question or brings up a concern, the issue is obviously important to him. We all respond best when we feel as though we are being heard. It is crucial, then, to use good listening skills when responding to questions. Let's look at some patient questions and how a dental professional might respond.

Patient: "I saw something on TV a couple of weeks ago about how metal fillings are really bad for you. Are you going to take out all of my metal fillings and replace them with safe ones?"

Dental Professional: "I saw that same report. This is a topic that dentists have been studying and discussing for quite a while. Our main goal in this office is to give you the best care possible, and part of that is to not do any treatment that isn't necessary."

Patient: "Well, that's good. But that one guy on the news had all of his fillings replaced, and he said that his health got much better afterwards."

Dental Professional: "Of course, you're in the driver's seat when it comes to the dental treatment we do, since they're your teeth.

There were some points that the news story didn't cover that suggest replacing all metal fillings isn't always the best idea. Would it be okay if I gave you some more information you can use to make your decision?"

In this example, the dental professional did not take a stand on either side of a controversial issue and did not dismiss the patient's concerns. Note that the dentist offered to provide information so that the patient could make an informed decision. It is important *not* to present information in a way that suggests, "I'm the expert, so this is what you need to do."

Patient: "My sister's friend said that she had an allergic reaction to the Novocain her dentist gave her. I don't want you giving me any of that!"

Dental Professional: "I can understand why you wouldn't want that to happen to you! Have you had something that felt like an allergic reaction to the local anesthetic that we used to numb your tooth before?"

Patient: "Well, no, but this woman hadn't had a reaction before, either.

Dental Professional: "I'm glad you brought up this concern to me. In the local anesthetic that we use, there's a chemical called epinephrine, which our bodies make naturally. It helps the local anesthetic last longer so that it doesn't wear off in the middle of filling a tooth."

Patient: "Well, I definitely don't want it to wear off! But are some people allergic to the stuff that's in the anesthetic?"

Dental Professional: "Some people may feel effects of the epinephrine more than others, but because it's something that our bodies make naturally, it's not really an allergic reaction. Some people may feel a little dizzy or their heart rate may go up a little, which makes them feel as though they're having an allergic reaction. While it may feel a little uncomfortable, there's no danger, and it passes quickly."

Patient: "So, my throat won't close up or anything?"

Dental Professional: "No, nothing like that. But we always keep a close eye on how you're doing, no matter what we're doing.

Would it be okay if we gave you a little bit of local anesthetic and see how you do with that? If you're not feeling okay after that, we'll wait until you're feeling better and then try some anesthetic that doesn't have epinephrine in it. That doesn't last as long, but if we decide to do a small filling today, it won't be a problem."

Patient: "That sounds like a good plan. Thanks."

Many patients come in for treatment having heard "horror stories" from other people. As with the previous example, it's important to validate patients' concerns and then provide information in appropriate terms. It is not helpful to use terms like "vasocontrictor" or "sympathetic arousal" with most patients, but you also want to avoid using terms that are too simple, particularly with adults.

Patient: "Both of my parents have lost almost all of their teeth. Why should I bother to get my teeth fixed now if they're just going to fall out?"

Dentist: "It makes sense that because of your parents' experiences, you expect that you will lose all of your teeth, too. One thing to keep in mind is that we have many more ways to keep teeth healthy than we had in the past, and many more treatments that can save teeth that would have been lost in your parents' time. If you are interested, we could talk about some of these today."

Patient: "Yeah. I really don't want to have dentures by the time I'm 45, like my dad did!"

In a case like this, it might be tempting to lecture patients, saying, "Well, if you take better care of your teeth than your parents did, you won't have to lose them." This approach will only make patients defensive, and any message you may want to get across will not be heard.

Non-Verbal Assessment of Health Literacy

We have already reviewed some of the kinds of questions patients may ask that can give you an idea of their health literacy. Some patients, however, particularly those with low levels of health literacy, find it difficult to know what questions to ask. These patients may prefer to take a more passive role in their oral health care and give complete control to the dental professional.

This passive approach may make individual appointments shorter due to a lack of questions. However, it is likely these patients will continue being passive in their oral health care at home. They may not follow the home care guidelines you suggest. This will lead to more oral problems in the future and further reinforce a feeling of helplessness.

Getting information across to passive patients may be more challenging than educating patients who ask many questions, because it is more difficult to assess what passive patients do and don't understand. Just because patients don't ask questions, though, doesn't mean they don't have any! With these patients, it is often helpful to ask open-ended questions to help get an idea of their knowledge and understanding.

What you should avoid:

Dental Professional: "Do you have any questions about what we're going to do today?"

Patient: "Nope."

Instead, you can say:

Dental Professional: "What do you remember about what we said we were going to do today?"

Patient: "I think we talked about filling that one tooth on top that's been hurting."

Dental Professional: "Right, that's what we had planned for today. If there are other teeth that are bothering you, though, we can talk about fixing those today instead."

Patient: "No, that's pretty much the only one. But I did notice that my gums are kind of swollen and puffy on the other side, too."

Dental Professional: "Okay. Thank you for letting me know about that. If it's okay with you, I'll go ahead and get that upper tooth numb and then take a look at your gums while we're waiting for the tooth to get numb."

Patient: "Sure, that sounds okay."

Open-ended questions encourage patients to voice their concerns and questions, rather than simply answering "yes" or "no." Open-ended questioning also demonstrates that you are focused on taking time to listen to their concerns, rather than simply getting through the procedure and on to the next patient.

It is also very important to assess a patient's understanding and knowledge whenever you introduce a new procedure or term into a treatment plan, particularly when patients do not ask questions. Don't assume that patients know what you are talking about! Most patients have had their teeth "cleaned" or a "cavity filled." However, when suggesting less routine treatments such as endodontic procedures, extractions, or periodontal treatment, it is good to stop and check in with patients about their prior experiences, understanding, and expectations.

What you should avoid:

Dental Professional: "So, after looking at your X-rays, I would probably suggest doing a root canal on number 2."

Patient: "Um, okay."

Instead, you can say:

Dental Professional: "Let me show you your X-rays. This tooth here (point to number 2) is on the upper right, the second one from the back. Can you feel that with your tongue?"

Patient: "Yeah, that's the one that's been hurting."

Dental Professional: "Right. If you look on this X-ray, does it look any different from the one next to it?"

Patient: "Yeah, it does. It looks like part of it is missing."

Dental Professional: "Right. That tooth has a pretty big cavity in it, and the cavity is down into the nerve in the center of the tooth, which is why it has been hurting. In the past, we may have taken this tooth out, but we have new ways today to keep teeth that have cavities in them like this one."

Patient: "I definitely want to keep the tooth if I can."

Dental Professional: "Great! We want you to keep your teeth, too! What I'd like to suggest is something called a root canal procedure. What do you think of when I say that?"

Patient: "Oh, no! I've heard terrible stories about those. You want to go in and rip the roots out of my tooth?"

Dental Professional: "No, I definitely don't want to do that! I know that root canals have had a really bad reputation in the past. But now we have a lot of different things we do so that it's really no different from having a regular cavity filled; it just takes a little bit longer. Is it okay if I tell you more about it so you can decide for yourself what you want to do?"

Patient-Friendly Terminology

In pediatric dentistry, great attention is paid to using "kid-friendly" terms such as "raincoat" for rubber dam and "sleepy juice" for local anesthetic. These terms are too simplistic for most adults, but terms that are too technical should also be avoided. The following are terms that will require little, if any, explanation for most adults. You should always be aware of your patients' individual levels of understanding and alter your language accordingly.

Dental Terminology	*Patient-Friendly*
Lidocaine, etc.	Local Anesthetic, "what people used to call Novocaine"
Endodontic treatment	Root Canal
Saliva ejector	Suction, "vacuum"
Extraction	Taking a tooth out, removing the tooth (note: avoid using the term "pulling")
Caries	Cavity, decay
Pain	Discomfort, pressure

In this example, the dental professional encouraged the patient to be an active participant in the discussion by translating the radiograph into a description of the painful tooth. The dental professional also assessed what the patient knew and felt about endodontic treatment by asking how the patient felt when presented with the term "root canal." The patient's concerns were validated, and then the she was reassured that the procedure was not as difficult she perceived. In addition, throughout the conversation, the dental professional used terminology that was not too simple or complex.

Summarizing Health Literacy in the Dental Office

As we've discussed, it is important to assess what patients know, how they've learned what they know, and how to use their knowledge and understanding to further educate them about oral health issues. Here are some basic skills to keep in mind as you assess patients' health knowledge:

Listen carefully to patients' questions. Do not discredit sources that may be less than fully reliable. Reinforce patients for seeking out information.

Listen to what patients aren't saying. Do not assume that just because patients aren't asking questions that they don't have questions! If a patient responds with only "yes" or "no," use more open-ended questions and listen for concerns and misunderstandings in their responses.

Validate patients' concerns. Even if you feel that concerns are unwarranted, they are valid to patients, and you should find the "kernel of truth" in the concern before giving reassurances.

Avoid empty reassurances. Be specific in your reassurances; for example, "Once your tooth is numb, you shouldn't feel any more discomfort. Please let me know if you do feel anything." Avoid broad statements like, "Everything is going to be okay."

Avoid "talking down" to patients. Just because a patient does not understand all of the dental jargon that is second nature in the dental field does not mean that he is not capable of understanding these concepts with slightly different terminology. However, you should avoid using terms that are too simplistic or childish. "Talking down" to patients gives the impression that you do not think they are intelligent individuals who are capable of deciding on their own dental care.

Maintain a constant flow of communication. Once a patient has been part of your practice for a period of time, it is easy to assume that he or she "just knows" what you mean. Be sure to check in with your patient from time to time to assure that you are both still "on the same page" with regard to treatment.

Satisfaction with Dental Care

What determines how satisfied people are with their dental care? Research using a measure called the Dental Satisfaction Questionnaire (DSQ) has found that the following factors are critical in assessing patients' satisfaction with their dental care:

Availability/convenience: This factor relates to the presence of a sufficient number of dentists in an area and how conveniently located these dentists are.

Access: This relates to how difficult it is to get a dental appointment and how long patients must wait once they arrive at the dental office.

Cost: As the term implies, this factor relates to how high a dentist's fees are and how much patients feel a dentist avoids unnecessary expenses.

Pain Management: This refers to patients' desire to avoid dentists who they perceive do not care about patients' pain and who cause pain. This also relates to wanting to seek out dentists who control pain.

Quality has also been found in some research to relate to satisfaction with dental care. This factor refers to such issues as a dentist's thoroughness in care, ability to relieve and prevent oral health problems, treating patients with respect, having a modern dental office, and explaining the purpose and cost of treatment effectively.

Finally, the simplest way to assess how satisfied your own patients are with their care is simply to ask them. *Debriefing* may be especially useful. A simple question at the end of an appointment, such as, "Tell me, how did it go?" may allow patients an avenue of communication that is not always available. As previously advised, avoid asking "yes or no" questions, and be open to any concerns that patients may have. Patients who feel that their dentists are willing to hear their concerns tend to be much more satisfied with their care than patients who feel that their concerns aren't heard.

A Few Words about Control

Research with both adults and children has shown that a large percentage of dental patients prefer to have some kind of control during dental treatment. In addition, many fearful dental patients note that they feel "out of control" while in the dental situation, in that they have no ability to stop the procedure if needed. There are a number of simple ways to help patients feel more in control in the dental setting.

Providing *informational control* to patients involves not just telling them the procedure that will be done that day, but also giving details about what they will feel (i.e., pressure, a "mosquito bite," etc.), for how long, and when. Patients who know that "something bad" is going to happen, but do not know when, remain in a constant state of anxiety. If patients know when to expect an aversive event, they will be able to feel more relaxed. You can use several techniques to signal aversive events for patients.

- "I'm going to use my drill for the count of three, then stop. When I stop, I'll take the drill out of your mouth, and you can tell me how that felt."
- "Right now, you're going to feel a slight pinch, then some pressure. Take a few deep breaths first, and let me know when you're ready."

Cognitive control refers to a patient's ability to change what he or she is thinking about a situation. Many fearful dental patients report that during dental treatment, they continually have very negative thoughts about the situation. This is called *catastrophizing*, in that a patient may feel that having dental work is definitely a catastrophe! For example, a patient may repeatedly think such things as, "This is terrible," "I can't stand another minute!" "This is going to be so painful." As a result, the patient's thoughts will lead to increased feelings of anxiety and tension during treatment.

You can help increase patients' cognitive control by suggesting that they think of other, calming things such as a favorite spot or a pleasant vacation in order to distract themselves from the dental setting. In addition, patients can replace their negative, catastrophizing thoughts with more positive coping statements. For example, patients can tell themselves, "This isn't so bad, I can get through this," "It will only last for a minute, I can handle it." By encouraging more positive statements, you can help patients feel more in control of their thoughts and emotions during treatment.

When telling patients about an aversive event that is about to happen, it is also important to suggest ways in which they can cope with the event. Deep, slow breathing, imagining themselves in a pleasant spot, and using the positive self-statements described above are all ways in which patients can actively cope with aversive events, rather than just passively "toughing it out."

Another important factor to consider is *how much* information patients want to have. Although many patients want to know what is happening and when, some patients would rather not know. Giving them explicit details about the procedure will only increase their anxiety. It is crucial to find out early on about the amount of information patients want to have. For example, during an initial examination you can say, "Some people like to know everything that's going on during treatment, but others don't want to know anything. What do you prefer?" If a patient states she does not want to know anything about what is going on, then you can suggest a number of distraction techniques, such as listening to music on headphones or imagining a pleasant scene. It is important to match a patient's desire for information with the type and amount of information you provide.

Retrospective control refers to reviewing patients' experiences *after* the appointment. As previously noted, *debriefing* can help patients establish a sense of control after the aversive event has happened. By asking "How did it go today?" you can help the patient identify areas of difficulty. For example, a patient may explain that he "started to freak out" during the injection. By asking more questions about this, you both may discover that not only was the patient catastrophizing (i.e., telling himself that the injection was going to be very painful), but that he felt physically ill because he held his breath during the injection. Identifying these factors after the fact will help the patient understand what made the injection difficult and allow him to use different skills during the next visit (i.e., using positive self-statements and deep breathing). Debriefing may also make the difference between a patient's not returning for care ("That really hurt") and the patient's returning ("It hurt, but we now have a plan so that I'll be more comfortable next time").

Barriers to Communication

We have described several general ways to communicate with your patients. Each patient, however, comes into your office with his or her own individual beliefs, experiences, and expectations regarding dental treatment. These individual factors need to be taken into account when you interact with your patients. The communication skills described throughout this book are important for all patients, but individual differences are just as important to consider in communicating effectively with patients.

Cultural Differences

When discussing how cultural differences affect perceptions of dental care, it is important to remember that the information provided here is not meant to serve as a precise description of each member of a cultural group. Every cultural group is heterogeneous, and dental professionals should be sensitive to individual differences within each group.

> You may find additional information regarding culturally specific dental care considerations on the EthnoDent web site at www.ethnodent.org.

Cultural differences may manifest themselves in the ways people utilize dental services, view the importance of preventive dental care, and interact with dental providers. For example, research with Mexican-American focus groups suggests that tooth decay is seen as a normal part of childhood, and that although good oral hygiene can lower the rate of childhood tooth decay, "baby teeth" are not seen as being as important as permanent teeth. Similar focus groups with Chinese-Americans found that the primary reason for utilizing dental services was to alleviate pain, rather than for preventive measures. In addition, members of these focus groups explained that they typically do not use toothbrushes with their children until the age of 3 or 4. Before that time, they typically use a cloth to wipe the child's teeth and have the child rinse his or her mouth with water.

Members of some cultural groups may speak with health providers without making eye contact. This should not be interpreted to mean that a patient is not listening to or interacting with providers. In some cultures, direct eye contact with a person in authority is seen as a sign of disrespect.

Taking time to listen to a patient's concerns is of utmost importance. When treating a patient from a different cultural background from your own, it is also important to keep in mind that this patient may view oral health very differently than you do. While you may not agree with the patient's view on oral health, it is crucial to respect this view while providing information on your perspective.

Experiences

Patients come to a dental office with a lifetime of dental experiences, both positive and negative. Regardless of your own technical expertise, communication skills, and chairside manner, you are faced with managing not only the experiences your patients have in your office, but also the experiences they have had with past dentists. Many patients will be more than willing to share their previous experiences with you, particularly if these experiences were negative.

- "My last dentist never listened to me. I told her it hurt, and she just kept drilling. I haven't been back since, and that was eight years ago."
- "The dentist I went to when I was a kid told me to stop being a

baby."

- "I loved my last dentist, and I was heartbroken when he retired. I don't think I'll ever find anyone who was as gentle as he was."

As with all discussions of communication skills, the first rule of thumb is to use good listening skills to show patients that you want to know about their past experiences and how you can either recreate their good experiences or avoid negative past events. Examples of questions and statements you can use are:

- "It sounds like you've had some difficult dental experiences in the past. Are there things that have been helpful for you in making dentistry easier (i.e., hand signals to stop, watching with a mirror, anti-anxiety medications, etc.)?"
- "I'm sorry that you had a bad experience with your last dentist, and we certainly don't want to repeat that here. What specific parts of dentistry to do you find most difficult (injections, drilling, rubber dams, etc.)?"
- "Your last dentist sounded great, and I'm sure it's hard for you to trust a new dentist. I'd like to talk more with you about what he did so well so that we know how you'd like to be treated. It will definitely take time for you to trust a new person, but I hope you and I can work on that together."

Even if the events a patient describes seem unbelievable to you, remember that these experiences are very real to the patient and should never be dismissed. Use general statements to acknowledge the patient's concerns and then focus the discussion on what you can do to make the patient comfortable now and in the future.

Patient: "I know I need to have my wisdom teeth out, but the last time I had a tooth pulled, the dentist didn't give me any Novocaine.... It was the most awful experience of my life."

Dental Professional: "I'm sorry that you had a very difficult experience in the past. Thank you for telling me about it. Now, I'd like to spend some time talking to you about what you would like to be different in our office."

Patient: "Yeah, because that last dentist was a butcher."

Dental Professional: "It sounds like in the past, your pain wasn't well-controlled. Let me tell you about the things we do here to make sure that you are comfortable..."

Note that in this scenario, the dental professional did not dwell on or dismiss the patient's prior experience, even if he or she doubted that the treatment happened exactly as the patient described it. When discussing difficult experiences with patients, the important factor is not what *actually* happened from a technical standpoint, but how the patient *perceived* what happened. Examples of what NOT to say are:

- "Oh, I'm sure it wasn't that bad."
- "I can't believe that a dentist didn't give you local anesthetic for that. Are you sure that's what happened?"
- "That doesn't sound right. You must be remembering that incorrectly."

The primary points to remember about addressing patients' prior experiences are to acknowledge them appropriately and focus on what you can do now and in the future to treat the patient well. Patients will appreciate the chance to tell their stories and talk about how to avoid future negative experiences.

Gender

No research has been done regarding patients' preferences for same- or opposite-gender dental providers. Some research in the medical literature suggests that female patients prefer same-gender providers, particularly in the area of obstetrics/gynecology. Results from these studies, however, have been mixed and do not necessarily translate to dentistry.

Issues related to patient gender, however, still need to be taken into consideration. For example, studies have suggested a positive relationship between dental fear and avoidance and sexual abuse history, at least for female patients. Many patients, however, do not report previous sexual abuse to their dental providers, and many practitioners do not inquire about such a history.

The key point in issues related to gender is to be sensitive. It is appropriate to ask all patients, regardless of history, if they would like to have a support person in the operatory with them during treatment. This support person may be a friend or family member, or could be a staff member. Patients often benefit from having "another pair of ears" to be part of the discussion and from having a supportive person in the operatory during treatment. It may be more common for female patients, particularly with an abuse history, to want a support person with them during treatment, but it should not be assumed that male patients or patients without an abuse history will not also benefit from the presence of a support person.

Physical Disabilities

Patients with physical disabilities may or may not have special considerations with regard to communicating with dental practitioners. For example, patients who are hearing-impaired may or may not be able to speak and/or read lips. If a hearing-impaired patient uses only sign language and no one in your practice is able to use or understand sign language, it is important for the patient to bring a friend or family member who may serve as a translator. The same is true if a patient is unable to speak for other reasons. This support person should remain in the operatory throughout the entire treatment session to assist in communication.

A patient who is blind or significantly visually impaired may not require a support person, but may require the dental provider to take additional time to explain treatment and help her navigate the dental office. A patient who is not visually impaired may need less in the way of beginning a procedure, as he is able to use visual cues to know when treatment is about to begin. When a patient is not able to use these visual cues, however, practitioners may use verbal cues. For example, you may say, "Mrs. Jones, is it okay for me to lean the chair back? Great. Now I'm going to ask you to open your mouth, and I'm going to use my mirror to look in your mouth." Of course, it is helpful to use such verbal cues with all patients, but it is particularly important for patients who are unable to use other sensory cues during treatment.

Some patients may present with physical disabilities, such as paraplegia, that make it difficult to sit in a dental chair for extended periods of time. The same communication skills should be used with these patients to gain information about their needs. Here are some examples:

- "Do you have any difficulties sitting for long periods of time? Would it be helpful to take breaks during treatment so you can readjust and be more comfortable?"
- "Do you need any help getting into or out of a dental chair? If so, would it be okay for our staff to help you, or would you prefer that a friend or family member help you?"
- "Is there anything else we can do to make you more comfortable?"

As previously mentioned, open-ended questions will allow you to gain more valuable information than "yes" or "no" answers.

Mental Health

In the United States, approximately 22 percent of adults have been diagnosed with some type of mental illness. It is likely, then, that you will have many patients in your practice with mental illness. To describe all the types of psychiatric diagnoses that you may encounter is outside the scope of this book, but we will present the diagnoses you are most likely to encounter and the general communication issues associated with these diagnoses.

Many people who have been diagnosed with a psychiatric disorder manage their symptoms effectively through medication and/or therapy, and any symptoms associated with their diagnosis will not significantly affect dental treatment. For example, patients diagnosed with major depression are often prescribed medications and may also work with a therapist. They may effectively manage their symptoms to the point that you would not identify anything different about them compared to non-depressed patients.

However, some psychiatric disorders, particularly if not treated, may interfere with dental care, particularly oral self-care at home. Examples of these are:

Panic Disorder: Patients with this type of anxiety disorder are highly attuned to physical sensations. For example, these patients dislike the sensation of topical and local anesthesia and may misinterpret these sensations as indicating that they are ill. Another example: a patient with Panic Disorder may feel that he cannot breathe when a rubber dam is placed, which could lead him to feel that he is suffocating, increasing his anxiety to the point of a full panic attack. In this case, the rubber dam should be removed and the patient encouraged to take slow, deep breaths until he feels calmer. Then treatment may continue at a slower pace, making sure that the patient understands the typical sensations associated with the procedure (i.e., pressure, tingling, etc.).

Fearful Patients

It is not uncommon for patients who fear dental treatment to have additional anxiety-related disorders. Skills used to manage any type of anxiety (e.g., deep breathing, muscle relaxation, guided imagery, distraction, etc.) can be used effectively with these patients. For more details about treating fearful patients in your practice, please refer to

Treating Fearful Dental Patients:
A Patient Management Handbook
by Milgrom, Weinstein and Getz (1995)

Mood Disorders: Among diagnoses in this category are major depression and bipolar disorder (previously called "manic-depression"). Patients with these disorders are unlikely to require special treatment in the dental office. However, one way mood disorders manifest themselves is through varying levels of motivation. Therefore, patients may at times have difficulty following through with treatment appointments and instructions for home care. Refer to the "Motivational Interviewing" chapter for a more thorough explanation of the role of motivation in oral self-care.

Mental Retardation: The American Psychiatric Association (APA) includes mental retardation (MR) in its diagnostic manual and defines MR in terms of varying degrees, from mild to profound. The impact of a patient's MR on receiving dental treatment and following through with oral self-care at home depends on the severity of the diagnosis. It is likely to be helpful to have a friend, family member, or caseworker in attendance during treatment planning and even during treatment, depending on the patient's individual needs. It is important to use terminology appropriate to the patient's intellectual functioning without "talking down" to her and assuming that she cannot understand information about treatment and self-care.

Many dental practitioners are uncomfortable addressing psychiatric diagnoses with patients, but because these diagnoses and their associated medications may affect dental treatment (e.g., many medications used to treat depression and anxiety cause xerostomia, or dry mouth, which in turn is a risk factor for caries), it is important to gain a full history, particularly during the initial session. Here is an example of how to start this conversation:

Dental Professional: "I see from your health history that you're currently taking (Prozac, Celexa, Zoloft, etc.). How long have you been taking that?"

Patient: "I don't know, a couple of years. My doctor prescribed it for me."

Dental Professional: "Has it been helpful for you?"

Patient: "Yeah, I guess. Why do you need to know about that?"

Dental Professional: "That's a good question. We ask all patients to tell us what medications they're taking, just to make sure that medications you use do not have an effect on your oral health or don't mix badly with the medicines we may recommend."

Patient: "Oh, okay. I'm just uncomfortable telling others about my problems."

Dental Professional: "I can understand your concerns, and I think it's great that you're taking steps to take care of yourself. Would it be okay with you if I checked in with you from time to time when you come in, just to be sure the medicine is still working? If not, then you can talk to your doctor about making some changes."

Patient: "Yeah, that would be okay."

Referring Patients for Further Treatment

At times, you may notice that a patient you've been treating for a period of time doesn't "seem like him/herself." The patient may seem quieter or more withdrawn, tearful, or anxious. A simple, non-judgmental statement such as, "How have you been feeling lately? You seem a little sad (jumpy, etc.) today." More often than not, patients will explain that they've been more stressed at work or tired because of a busy schedule.

Sometimes, though, a patient will reveal that he has been feeling much more sad or anxious than usual for a significant period of time. It is a good idea to keep a list of general mental health resources and/or specific names of therapists to give to patients. You may also suggest that he contact his primary care physician or insurance company for names of therapists. This conversation does not need to be extensive or involve a lot of "leg work" on the dental professional's part.

Dental Professional: "How have you been feeling lately? You seem pretty down in the dumps today."

Patient: "Yeah, I just don't know what's wrong. I'm crying all the time, I can barely drag myself out of bed in the morning, and I don't have any appetite."

Dental Professional: "That sounds really difficult, and I'm sorry you're having such a tough time right now. I have the names of some people that may be able to help you sort out what's going on. Would it be okay if I gave that list to you?"

Patient: "Well, I don't think I need to see a shrink or anything, if that's what you're saying."

Dental Professional: "No, I think we all go through times when we don't feel quite like ourselves, and sometimes it's helpful to talk to someone impartial to help us sort out what's going on. How about this... I'll give you the list of names, and you can do with it what you want. You're not obligated to call anyone just because you have the list. How does that sound?"

Patient: "Yeah, I guess that's okay. I can always hold on to the list if I need it later."

Conflict Resolution

Despite our best attempts to maintain good communication, it is inevitable that misunderstandings occur with some patients. Previously, we discussed factors that contribute to patients' satisfaction with dental treatment. Many conflicts that arise relate to these factors. Here are some examples of potential conflicts and solutions in the common areas of access, availability, cost, and pain management:

Problem: A patient becomes frustrated when she is unable to schedule an appointment that works with her hectic schedule (access).

Solution: If possible, reschedule another patient with a more flexible schedule (and agreeable temperament!) on one occasion so the first patient may have the first or last appointment of the day. Explain to the first patient that although you are not usually able to adjust times, you understand about hectic schedules and will work around hers when possible.

Problem: A patient expresses annoyance that he has to drive many miles out of his way to come to your office (availability).

Solution: Agree that there is a shortage of dental providers in the area (if there is) and that you can schedule longer appointments to get more treatment done so that he does not have to travel as often.

Problem: A patient complains that her treatment is too expensive (cost).

Solution: Validate (agree with) her concerns about cost and, if possible, arrange for her to make manageable payments on a regular basis. You can also schedule treatments across a longer period of time.

Problem: A patient refuses to pay his outstanding balance (cost).

Solution: Discuss the reason for his refusal to pay. If finances are an issue, set up a payment plan that works with his monthly budget. If he states that unnecessary treatment was done, remind him that he previously agreed to the proposed treatment plan. Make it clear to him that no further treatment will be done until the balance is paid. Remind him of the payment plan and, if possible, readjust payments.

Problem: A patient calls to cancel an appointment, saying that when she was in the last time, she felt a lot of pain during her cleaning and doesn't want to come back (pain management).

Solution: Phone the patient and tell her that you're sorry she felt pain during her last appointment, and that it's always your goal for your patients to be comfortable. Offer to reschedule the next appointment and meet with her prior to the appointment to talk about how you can better control her pain. Include the use of hand signals to stop the procedure at any time and the use of local and topical anesthetics (see Milgrom, Weinstein, and Getz, 1995).

Many complaints brought up by dental patients are related to the cost of treatment. However, disagreements about cost may mask patients' real concerns. For example, if a patient feels as though his concerns were not heard or considered by the dental staff, he is likely to leave the office feeling upset or angry. Rather than stating his real concerns (which he may or may not be able to identify), he may make statements such as, "I can't believe you charge so much for that." Ask open-ended questions such as, "It sounds like you have some concerns about the treatment we did today. How do you feel that it went?" Open ended questions encourage patients to describe not only the technical side of treatment, but allow them to express their subjective experiences. For example, this patient may respond, "Well, it was all going okay until about halfway through, but then it started to hurt and I didn't want to say anything." Encouraging patients to express their real concerns enhances their satisfaction with care.

Conclusion

Good communication with patients is just as important as technical ability and having the most up-to-date equipment in your office. You may perform a technically near-perfect dental procedure, but if the patient does not feel as though you have listened to his concerns and done your best to understand his needs, it is not likely that he will return or refer friends or family members to your practice. Dental professionals should always take individual differences into account while using good communication skills with each patient. Differences in culture, experiences, gender, physical disabilities, and psychiatric diagnoses all can present unique challenges with regard to communication. By using the skills presented in this chapter, dental professionals can establish rapport with patients that will minimize conflict and help ensure patient satisfaction with their dental care.

Assignments for Chapter 2

The following vignettes are meant to demonstrate some of the interactions with patients who you may encounter. They require you to use your best communication skills. If possible, role-play these vignettes with your classmates or colleagues, practicing what you would say in situations like these.

Assignment 1:

Your new patient, Mr. G, is a 54-year-old man with good periodontal health and moderate posterior caries. When you tell him he will need several fillings to restore his oral health to a good condition, he responds that both of his parents had lost all of their teeth by the time they were his age. He says that rather than "go to all the trouble of having those teeth filled," he would prefer to have all his teeth extracted and have full dentures made. After consulting his x-rays and your colleagues, it is your belief that he would benefit more from having restorations and keeping his teeth for many more years.

- What are the barriers to keeping all of his teeth, from the Mr. G's point of view? What are the benefits that he sees to having his teeth extracted and receiving full dentures?

- How do you relate to Mr. G that you understand his point of view?
- What are the benefits you see for Mr. G if he keeps his teeth? What barriers do you see?
- How will you present this information to Mr. G? Keep in mind that you do not want to "blame" his parents for losing their teeth. Instead, consider what changes have been made in dentistry in recent years that give Mr. G more choices than his parents may have had.
- If Mr. G remains certain that he wants all of his teeth extracted, how will you feel about following through with this treatment plan?

Assignment 2:

You have been seeing Mrs. P for 3 years, and although she expressed some anxiety about having dental treatment done when you first started seeing her, she says that she has come to trust you and no longer fears having dental work done in your office. During one particular treatment session, you noticed that Mrs. P had been more "fidgety" than usual and seemed somewhat uncomfortable at times. You asked her if she was uncomfortable or in pain, and she said she was "fine." However, after finishing the procedure, you notice that Mrs. P is not as talkative as usual, and she leaves in somewhat of a hurry. Mrs. P then misses her next scheduled appointment. When your office manager calls to reschedule her appointment, Mrs. P becomes angry, saying she was "overcharged" for her last treatment. You decide to call Mrs. P to discuss her concerns.

- How do you start the conversation? What do you want to know from this patient?
- During the conversation, Mrs. P suggests that she is not very upset about the cost of the treatment, but that she "just didn't feel right about how things went" during the procedure. What questions do you ask to find out more about Mrs. P's concerns?
- After asking more questions about the procedure, you realize that Mrs. P was feeling pain but was "embarrassed" to tell you. What do you say?

- What would do want the outcome of this conversation to be? How do you relate this to Mrs. P? How can you make Mrs. P's next visit to you a more positive one?

Assignment 3:

You are seeing a 4-year-old patient for the first time. She and her parents immigrated from Mexico 18 months ago, and her mother, Mrs. A, brought her in to see you because she is having pain in one of her "baby" teeth. Mrs. A also brought a neighbor, Ms. F, who speaks English well, to translate. You notice that your patient has extensive caries, and you ask Mrs. A, through Ms. F's translation, about how she takes care of her daughter's teeth. Mrs. A reports that although she brushes her daughter's teeth once a day, she often gives her soft drinks and sugary snacks during the day. Mrs. A says that in their community, all kids have cavities, and that tooth pain is not uncommon. She tells you that because her daughter will lose these teeth soon anyway, she does not understand why you are suggesting that she have her cavities filled.

- How do you address your concerns about your patient's oral health while avoiding judgmental statements about her diet and oral health habits?
- How do you explain to Mrs. A why you feel it is important to fix her daughter's "baby" teeth?
- What else would you want to know about Mexican culture to better understand this family's beliefs?

The unfortunate thing about this world is that good habits are so much easier to give up than bad ones.

S. Maugham

It isn't that they can't see the solution. It is that they can't see the problem.

G. K. Chesterton

Chapter 3

Therapeutic Alternatives

This chapter contains many references to research articles about the effectiveness of various kinds of fluoride, toothbrushes, and other oral care products. By nature of the topic, you will likely find this chapter to be more technically-oriented than many of the others in this book. For additional information about the products discussed here, please refer to the reference section at the end of the book.

It is frustrating to encounter a patient whose oral health problem could be addressed by better home care but who is unable or unwilling to change or to adopt new behaviors. Such a situation requires long-term behavioral solutions. However, short-term therapeutic alternatives are also needed; that is, the clinician must expend greater professional effort in lieu of patient action.

Why can't you just insist that the patient follow your recommendations? After all, it is in the patient's best interest. If Mary does not improve her hygiene, all her new restorative work will fail. Tom will develop caries around his orthodontic brackets and we'll have to remove the appliances.

The reality is that patients have choices too, and the "my way or the highway" approach rarely leads to better adherence to instructions. Adults may simply avoid follow-up appointments or leave the practice. Teens will become sullen and uncommunicative. In this type of situation, staff members burn out and quit or become afraid to bring up the touchy subject with their supervisors. They often ineffectively threaten youngsters with parental intervention, which leads to loss of rapport and rarely to long-term cooperation.

The key to success is providing many choices. If a patient takes little or no responsibility for home care, for whatever reason, the clinician may assume more responsibility. Over time, as rapport develops between patient and practice, the patient is likely to engage in treatment and take greater responsibility. The timeline varies among patients, and there is no set rule. In the meantime, everyone works within his or her capacity to maintain and improve health.

This chapter is organized in order of five important steps. These steps are similar to the behavior change strategies presented in more detail later in the book. The steps covered in this chapter, however, focus primarily on the introduction of different therapeutic alternatives that may be later incorporated into a larger behavior change program. The five steps covered in this chapter are:

1: Identify the problem and ascertain the patient's willingness to consider alternatives.

2: Consider the alternatives to be proposed.

3: Specify goals of the strategy, figuring out specific and realistic intermediate and terminal objectives.

4: Plan and implement procedures and strategy.

5: Monitor and troubleshoot.

Identify the Problem

Problems vary widely. An uncooperative adolescent patient refuses to brush her teeth and is developing caries. Another patient breaks his arm and has temporary trouble maintaining adequate oral cleanliness. Each patient is at risk for starkly different reasons. The clinician's task at this stage is to gather information about the specific problem and to use interviewing skills to gauge the patient's willingness to consider alternatives. We might assume that the alternatives for these two patients will differ widely.

Consider the Alternatives

Keeping the problem(s) of a specific patient in mind, the clinician can consider alternative treatments. We can begin by reviewing basic cariology. Human teeth, when colonized by mutans streptococci and lactobacillus, are damaged by lactic acid produced as part of the metabolism of the bacteria. The bacteria are part of the human tooth biofilm, or plaque, and are usually a small proportion of the oral bacterial community. However, in patients with diets high in carbohydrates or in patients with lots of fillings or prosthetic or orthodontic appliances, the proportion of "bad actors" increases. Lactic acid diffuses through the outer white enamel of the tooth and damages the dentin, or less calcified layer, below. Next, the crystalline enamel structure fails and falls in. This is a cavity. Often in an initial occlusal cavity, the damaged area under the enamel is larger than the enamel defect on the surface. The initial occlusal lesion begins on the smooth vertical walls of the occlusal grooves just as it does on other surfaces of the teeth. This is also true for interproximal cavities; the initial damage is to the underlying dentin, even though it appears as if the bacteria are drilling their way from the outside in.

The early stage of a tooth lesion is called a "white spot" and is always reversible. It is white because light passes through the enamel differently than through an area where the tooth is intact. The lesions are often white but may also appear yellow or even brown. Effective action taken at this stage will always prevent a full-blown cavity. In the Appendix, there are caries risk assessment forms that include recommendations on the steps to take for both children and adults. Patients in professional care with "white spot" lesions should never be allowed to develop cavities simply because their oral hygiene is inadequate. This represents a failure to utilize any or all of the following therapeutic alternatives:

Topical Fluoride Varnish. Topical fluoride varnish is used to arrest and remineralize damaged tooth structure before cavitation can occur. "White spot" lesions are often seen in the cervical third of the clinical crown. Varnish is also effective in arresting already cavitated lesions, even when there is visible involvement of the dentin. Varnish is the most effective and quickest way to administer topical fluoride in the dental office and is widely available. It is the only form of professionally delivered topical fluoride that is safe and effective for preschoolers. Intervening at or before the white spot stage is an important professional alternative.

Because they are more effective, fluoride varnishes have largely replaced gels and trays in Europe and other parts of the world. Varnishes are slowly being adopted in the United States and Canada. They were developed in the 1960s in Europe based on varnishes that previously were placed under amalgam fillings and were used to reduce tooth sensitivity. At least five different fluoride varnishes are sold in the United States, and all of them follow the same basic formula as the original cavity varnish, *Duraphat*® (Colgate Oral Pharmaceuticals). Other varnishes popular with dental offices are *Duraflor*® (Pharmascience, Inc.) and *Cavity Shield*® (OMNII Oral Pharmaceuticals). Some of the products come as multi-use tubes; others come as single unit systems. Convenience generally dictates the choice.

Fluoride varnish is also used by public health nurses and physicians in many parts of the United States and Canada as part of an effort to improve the oral health of high-risk children. Fluoride varnish is a covered benefit under Medicaid in most states. Fluoride varnish is approved by the U.S. Food and Drug Administration. Fluoride varnish may be applied by dental hygienists and dental assistants working under indirect or general supervision.

In adults and older children, fluoride varnish is applied by first drying the teeth with gauze, a quadrant at a time, and then applying a layer of varnish with a small applicator such as a *Kwik Tip* ™. Fluoride varnish sets on contact with moisture, so it is unnecessary to have a completely dry field. After each application, the varnish should be flossed between the teeth. It can be placed on both smooth and fissured surfaces. A prophylaxis is not needed before the application of fluoride varnish. Fluoride varnish works by establishing a depot for fluoride in the fluid layer of the biofilm, or plaque. Fluoride is released from the biofilm to do its job when bacterial acids lower the pH at the tooth surface. Applying fluoride varnish is so quick that our staff works these patients in between other scheduled appointments. It takes only a minute or two to provide the service.

Fluoride varnish has a dose-effect relationship; that is, applying fluoride more often increases its cavity prevention effect. Twice per year application, in teens for example, has been shown to reduce new cavities by about one-third compared to brushing with fluoride toothpaste alone. Three times per year is more effective. Many practices and insurers in the United States have adopted a bi-annual regimen for topical fluoride. A thinking clinician will adapt this approach to the situation he or she faces.

Another alternative is repeated application of fluoride varnish several times in a two- or three-week period, which studies show might be as effective as one application every six months. This alternative may be helpful in situations such as those faced by clinics serving migrant workers or other mobile or transient populations, in which it may be difficult to recall an adult or child for follow-up fluoride application.

For babies or preschoolers, the application regimen is modified based on the cooperation level of the child. Many children in this age range may complain or cry, although this represents an unwillingness to be restrained rather than pain or discomfort. Fluoride varnish does not sting, and its taste to a child is neutral. The knee-to-knee approach is best. Parent and clinician sit in two facing chairs. The child lies with legs around the parent's waist and head in the clinician's lap. The parent can help restrain the child's arms and hands. Tilt the head up so that it is relatively easy to visualize the teeth. Experienced clinicians use a toothbrush as a mouth prop. Before applying the varnish, always do a visual inspection. With a single operator-clinician, it is best to place a glob of the varnish on one of the gloved hands, leaving the hands free to manipulate gauze and the applicator. With two operators, it is possible to have the second hold the varnish container and pass the applicator. In this case, the teeth are dried as thoroughly as possible (upper and lower separately) and the fluoride applied. It is rarely a perfect application as is possible on adults' teeth, but evidence suggests it works just the same. Again, a prophylaxis is not needed prior to a fluoride treatment. If there is a lot of food debris in the child's mouth, a toothbrushing beforehand may be appropriate.

Fluoride varnish does not stain teeth. However, parents should be advised that with the typical fluoride varnish a brownish film on the teeth may remain for a day or so and that the temporary discoloration is normal. At least one commercial producer of varnish is now marketing a white varnish that may be useful for patients who are sensitive to the color of the typical varnish.

Safety of Fluoride Varnish

After fluoride varnishes became popular because of their caries preventive action, their high concentration of fluoride made it necessary to evaluate the risk of possible side effects. Ekstrand *et al.* (1980) investigated the plasma F levels in 4 children after oral application of Duraphat®. In this study, 0.11-0.15 ml of Duraphat® was applied to younger children's teeth (supplying a dose of 2.3-3.0 mg). Older children received 0.25 ml varnish containing 5.0-5.2 mg F. The highest plasma fluoride concentration varied between 60 and 120 ng F/ml and was seen within 2 hours of application. These values are far below those considered toxic (Cousins & Mazze, 1973). For nonrenal toxicity, the amount of swallowed Duraphat® or other varnish necessary to exceed the "probably toxic dose" for fluoride (5 mg/kg) would be 2.5 ml and 5 ml, respectively, in 10-kg and 20-kg children (Whitford, 1996). Therapeutic applications are far below these doses.

Observational case reports have provided other information regarding Duraphat's® side effects. Isaksson *et al.* (1993) reported on two cases of contact allergy to Duraphat®. They found that a skin-sensitizing rosin (colophony) is present in Duraphat®. The first case revealed that a dental nurse with a history of hand eczema had sensitivity to Duraphat®. Patch testing with Duraphat® yielded a strong positive reaction in this case. The In the second case, a person who received Duraphat treatments developed edema of the tongue, soft palate, and upper lip within 24 h of receiving the treatment. The patient also showed positive reactions to separate patch tests with Duraphat® and colophony. Isaksson and others found no other reports in the literature on contact stomatitis or contact dermatitis due to Duraphat® exposure. They suggest that patients "already hypersensitive to colophony can acquire allergic contact stomatitis from Duraphat®."

The only report that addresses hypersensitivity due to the active ingredient in Duraphat®, sodium fluoride, is by Camarasa, Serra-Baldrich, Lluch and Malet (1993). They reported on a case of contact urticaria in a young girl who had received a topical application of Duraphat®. She experienced "a very severe disseminated acute urticaria and facial angiodema" and required hospital admission. Further information showed that the girl had a history of being intolerant to certain fluoride toothpastes.

A third study used questionnaires to assess side effects to dental hygienists' treatment (Hensten-Petersen & Jacobsen, 1994). Although hygienists reported more side effects from Duraphat® in young children, this was probably due to the fact that the topical varnish is applied more predominantly in this age group. Some of the side effects reported were sickness, nausea, vomiting, itching hands and arms, perioral urticaria, gingival itch, and swelling of respiratory mucosa. The majority of observations reported sickness, nausea, and vomiting as the nature of the side effects, while perioral urticaria and gingival itch were single observations only.

In conclusion, sodium fluoride varnish contains fluoride in amounts far below those necessary to cause acute toxicity. Although applications may cause hypersensitivity in some people, the cases are rare. Even though sensitivity is rare, a complete medical history of the patient and the use of gloves by the clinician are called for.

Some offices and public health programs have been reluctant to adopt fluoride varnish because in the United States the products are not labeled for caries control. However, the dental products industry has been unwilling, at least to date, to expend the huge amounts of money required to convince the FDA that the labeling should be changed. Nevertheless, use of fluoride varnish for caries control is legal and increasingly practiced.

Frequent Coronal Polish and Topical Fluoride Varnish. There is good evidence for the effectiveness of bimonthly professional coronal polish in conjunction with the application of fluoride varnish and interproximal flossing to prevent and control dental caries in children and adults. Depending on the laws and customs in each area, these treatments can be provided by dental hygienists or specially trained dental assistants. Studies supporting the effectiveness of this approach stretch back more than 30 years (Axelsson, Nystrom, & Linde, 2004).

This polish and fluoride approach can be used in private practice or community health center dental programs but is especially effective in school-based systems of care where access to children or teens is easier. It can also be effective with the elderly, particularly in institutional living situations. It was pioneered by Professor Per Axelsson in Sweden but has been used in several countries, including Brazil, where caries rates are very high.

The technique uses low abrasive fluoride-containing polishing paste. It is based on the idea that it takes about two weeks for initial caries lesions to form in the teeth and that thorough professional plaque control bimonthly sufficiently disrupts the plaque biofilm to prevent serious damage to the teeth. Flossing is important for disrupting the biofilm interproximally, where many lesions form in the posterior teeth. Professional toothcleaning and individualized instruction have been shown to be effective, and the addition of topical fluorides to the regimen makes them more effective (Zickert, Lindvall & Axelsson,1982).

Dental flosses available in some parts of the world contain stannous fluoride or even antimicrobials. At present there is little evidence these products provide value-added to the basic technique of frequent professional tooth cleaning.

Chlorhexidine. Some patients, particularly those in orthodontic appliances, may benefit from professional application of chlorhexidine varnishes, rinses, or gels in addition to topical fluoride varnish and prophylaxis. This approach will lead to reduced tooth decay and to healthier gums (Axelsson, Paulander, Nordkvist & Karlsson, 1987; Axelsson, Lindhe, 1987). Some of the better products are not for sale in the United States but are available in other countries. Rinses, such as 0.12% chlorhexidine gluconate are available in the U.S., labeled as Peridex® (Omnii Oral Pharmaceuticals) or Perioguard®(Colgate Oral Pharmaceuticals). If applied once a day for two weeks every few months these rinses reduce *mutans streptococci* dramatically. Chlorhexidine used by itself in a home care regimen is unlikely to be effective in controlling dental caries.

Fluoride and chlorhexidine have different but compatible mechanisms of action. Fluoride primarily remineralizes teeth; chlorhexidine is an anti-microbial. Chlorhexidine helps reduce the level of *mutans streptococci* in the mouth. Fluoride toothpaste should not be used at the same time of day as chlorhexidine rinses because the detergents in the toothpaste may inactivate the chlorhexidine. Otherwise the use of both is compatible.

Chlorhexidine varnish (1% chlorhexidine/thymol, Cervitec® (Ivoclar Vivadent Ltd.)) has not been shown to be effective against dental caries and requires a particularly sensitive technique to apply (Plotzitza, Kneist, Berger & Hetzer, 2005). The varnish, applied to occlusal surfaces, has not been shown to alter mutans levels in other sites (Twetman & Petersson, 1998).

Some of the over-the-counter mouth rinses containing essential oils may reduce supragingival plaque and gingivitis if used regularly. For patients with gingivitis, subgingival irrigation with 10% povidone iodine in conjunction some professional tooth cleaning may be effective.

High Fluoride Toothpaste. Caries protection increases in relationship to the concentration of fluoride in toothpaste. Almost all toothpastes in the United States contain fluoride and are effective. *Toothpaste is more effective if patients abstain from rinsing with water right after brushing.* Some paste-gels, available by prescription, contain levels of fluoride up to 5,000 PPM, or almost five times that in normal toothpaste. An example is Prevident 5000® (Colgate Oral Pharmaceuticals). Some patients may be willing to change toothpastes. If gingivitis is a problem in addition to caries, use of a triclosan-containing toothpaste, such as Colgate Total® (Colgate-Palmolive Co.), may be useful. Parental supervision of toothbrushing in children increases its effectiveness.

We recommend high fluoride toothpaste whenever self care is less than optimal. At least when the patient does brush, more fluoride is delivered. High fluoride toothpaste can be prescribed for teenagers. *Its use in younger children requires parental monitoring to avoid overdoses.* High fluoride toothpaste is also recommended for school programs in which brushing under supervision is likely to bring down very high tooth decay rates.

The use of all toothpaste is more certain when it is mailed home or dispensed at the dental office on a regular basis. The service reduces barriers to access.

Exposure to Fluoridated Water. Don't forget to ask about the water that a patient is consuming. Both children and adults may be drinking bottled water without fluoride or may be filtering their water in a manner that removes fluoride. If a patient is having difficulty accomplishing home care, consumption of fluoridated water will help.

It is important for families to problem solve about water. If the water supply in their area is fluoridated but the family is not drinking from it, why? Is it taste, concerns about the safety of fluoride, lack of knowledge? Maybe it's just the convenience of the small water bottles. Suggest they fill the bottles from the supermarket with tap water or choose bottled water that contains fluoride. Do a little market research to see what is available. It is good to have examples in the office to show the patient or parent. Consider preparing a handout with local information that would help the family identify appropriate products.

It is difficult to give general guidelines for choosing water filters. The American Dental Association has tested various filters and concluded that some designs remove fluoride and others do not. Reverse osmosis and distillation techniques remove significant amounts of fluoride. Results for carbon filters vary. If a family is hooked on a particular system, encourage them to obtain a sample and have it tested locally. Most large communities and all states have accessible mechanisms for water testing.

Xylitol. Patients with orthodontic or removable prosthetic appliances, those with xerostomia (dry mouth), and others with poor hygiene may benefit from xylitol-containing toothpastes or from xylitol chewing gums or lozenges (Ly, Rothen & Milgrom, 2006). Only a few toothpastes contain 10 percent xylitol in addition to fluoride, which produces better caries control than fluoride toothpaste alone. Examples of xylitol-fluoride toothpastes available in the United States without prescription are Crest® Multicare Cool Mint (Procter & Gamble; be careful because other Crest® pastes do not contain significant amounts of xylitol) or Biotene® "Dry Mouth" toothpaste (Laclede). Epic also makes a xylitol/fluoride paste. These pastes tend to be expensive, so it is worth price shopping. Gums or other confections should list xylitol as the first active ingredient. *Exposures of at least 6 grams per day divided over at least three doses are needed to be effective.* When choosing among alternatives on the menu of choices for improving oral health, some individuals—particularly those who already chew gum—may find xylitol a doable approach. In the past, xylitol gums have been quite expensive, but the market is enlarging and the prices are dropping. Examples of gums containing effective amounts of xylitol are Hershey's® Carefree Koolerz™ gum, Lotte Xylitol gum, Epic Xylitol gum and Fenobon Xyli-Max gum. Since a xylitol habit can cost a dollar per day in 2006 dollars, price shopping is worthwhile.

Glass Ionomer or Composite Resin Sealants. For high risk but uncooperative patients or those who have difficulty adhering to home care, molars and/or premolars may be sealed. Typical BIS-GMA sealants require a dry field and scrupulous technique. Thus they are limited to situations where teeth are fully erupted and patients can tolerate careful isolation and drying. A new advance is the development of glass ionomer sealant materials that are not so moisture sensitive and can be placed on erupting teeth. Little has been published about this approach, but new techniques that may be effective are emerging. This topic is beyond the scope of this text, but many authoritative references are available.

Atraumatic Restorative Treatment. Fluoride-releasing glass ionomer filling materials can often be used without local anesthesia and drilling to temporize and arrest caries in patients whose caries disease is out of control or who cannot or will not cooperate with regular care. These tooth-sparing procedures allow professional intervention without huge amounts of patient follow through. High-strength materials, such as Ketac-Molar™ (3M), may be especially effective. Fuji IX™ and similar products release fluorides and may be recharged. It is remarkable how these cements function to arrest caries, both in primary and permanent teeth.

A very important application of ART is in permanent posterior teeth with deep decay on the occlusal aspect and invading dentin. Conventionally, a large prep is made and the damaged dentin removed completely with burs and spoons. In the ART approach, a smaller prep is made. Next, only the superficial damaged dentin is removed in order to create a mechanical undercut. Then the tooth is filled with glass ionomer. In most cases the caries process will arrest and the tooth will be less likely to fracture in the future because the preparation spares much tooth structure.

ART does not have to be 100 percent effective to be worth learning about and using. Some atraumatic restorations will come loose, but these can be replaced easily.

Fluoride Releasing Orthodontic Cements. Some evidence suggests that fluoride-releasing orthodontic cements may be superior to others in helping control caries. Most will be more effective only in conjunction with other professional activities such as topical fluoride varnish treatments (Benson, Shah, Millett, Dyer, Parkin & Vine, 2005).

Rotary and Ultrasonic Toothbrushes. Overall, there is no convincing body of evidence that these alternatives to standard toothbrushes are more effective than manual brushes for the general public. Nevertheless, some of the devices include timers and other cues to more effective brushing, and they may be effective in for some individuals. Their novelty may also increase utilization. They may or may not be more effective than other adaptive devices for the disabled or elderly. All such devices are best introduced under supervision.

Alternatives to Toothbrushes. Our clinical experience leads us to the conclusion that toothbrushes are hard for many patients to use consistently and effectively. Many will brush for only seconds. We have found that teens will adopt Stimudents® (Johnson & Johnson) or plain toothpicks for interdental cleaning even though they use the toothbrush infrequently. As with other aids, dispensing the toothpicks is likely to increase their application. In the "Teaching Skills" chapter we discuss the skill training needed to teach patients home care skills.

Silver Diamine Fluoride. This topical solution ($Ag(NH_3)_2F$, 38,000 PPM fluoride) is very effective in arresting cavitated lesions in teeth and preventing future tooth decay (Saforide, J. Morita Corporation, Osaka, Japan). It is useful in treating children too young to have restorative procedures or for primary teeth that will naturally exfoliate and are not abscessed, for children on waiting lists for treatment, and even for treating recurrence. It may be useful for treating elderly patients who cannot maintain good hygiene and do not have aides or family members who can help them.

Chu and colleagues (2002) studied the effect of diamine silver fluoride (SDF) in 375 preschool children, all having caries into the dentin in at least one of their upper primary anterior teeth. After a baseline examination, the children were divided randomly into four treatment groups and a placebo control. Group 1 had the soft dentin in the caries lesions removed by hand instruments then painted with 3.8% silver diamine fluoride solution (Saforide, J. Morita Corporation,

Osaka, Japan). Group 2 had Saforide solution applied every 12 months without excavation of carious dentin. Group 3 and Group 4 had 5% sodium fluoride (Duraphat, Inpharma GmbH, Cologne, Germany) painted on the lesions with and without removal of carious tissue respectively. For Group 5, a water control was painted on the carious tooth.

In groups 1-5, the percentages of arrested caries were 100%, 100%, 26%, 66%, and 42% respectively. Group 1, with the caries excavated and SDF applied, and Group 2, without the caries excavated and SDF applied, were the same, and both treatments provided a higher proportion of teeth with caries arrested than groups 3, 4, and 5. In all groups, no side effects were observed. Silver fluoride was more effective than either fluoride varnish or the placebo in preventing new lesions. The results were consistent with previous work by others (Nishino *et al.*, 1969; Moritani *et al.*, 1970; Yamaga *et al.*, 1972; Li, 1984). The proposed mechanism of action is via the formation of a silver phosphate layer on the tooth surface that is insoluble (Yamaga *et al.*, 1972). The dramatic preventive effect on other teeth may be a result of the fluoride in the lesions serving as a depot for fluoride release to other areas.

The primary safety issue with SDF is the potential for fluoride toxicity and fluorosis. Only a single laboratory study (Gotjamanos, 1997) addresses this issue, and its methods have been questioned (Neesham, 1997). This study suggested that 3 to 4 mg of fluoride would reach the systemic circulation after application of 40% silver fluoride solution from the product (available in Australia). Li and colleagues (1984) recommend a single annual application to minimize risk of fluorosis. The other criticism of SDF is that it turns the carious lesions black and therefore may be cosmetically objectionable.

The issues of fluorosis and lesion darkening are not of great importance in treating root caries. In adult and elderly patients, an application once or twice per year is effective in augmenting whatever efforts are made at home. The use of silver fluoride carries none of the compliance issues that plague home use of fluoride.

Anecdotally, there has been concern that silver fluoride may cause abscesses in primary teeth. It is likely that the on some teeth that would have abscessed in a this risk is unknown but is not, in our opinion, a valuable tool.

Silver fluoride products are available in Japan an possible for dentists to have silver fluoride compounde States and other countries where it is not available comm ly.

Specify Goals

It is axiomatic that getting a reluctant patient to take an initial step presages future cooperation. Often our goals are too lofty and extensive to be implemented immediately. Especially with patients having difficulty adhering to home care regimens, we need to present alternatives and ask the patient to choose an initial step. In our experience, more frequent visits—for services such as professional tooth cleaning and fluoride treatment—are the strategy of choice. Remember that this is an alternative to home care. Over time the situation of a patient will change and other alternatives can be pursued, based on the patient's readiness. Emphasis should be on repeated brief visits, often with no formal appointment required. For teens and children, appointments should be after school to minimize disruption to the school day and improve compliance with appointments.

All clinicians should be familiar with the Caries Risk Assessment recommended in the February and March 2003 issues of the California Dental Association Journal (Featherstone *et al.*, 2003). Forms for the risk assessment are included as an appendix to this book. The complete consensus statement by world experts is available free via the internet from the California Dental Association Foundation (www.cdafoundation.org). Using the Caries Risk Assessment approach allows a skilled clinician to assess how much effort is required to control tooth decay. Similarly, a periodontal disease assessment system is available commercially (www.previser.com) that maybe helpful to many clinicians and patients (Persson, Mancl, Martin & Page, 2003).

What do to for a reluctant teen

An initial goal for a reluctant or "precontemplative" teen with cervical demineralization in the lower cuspids and premolars might be bi-weekly application of topical fluoride varnish to the involved teeth (Milgrom, Rothen, Spadafora, Skaret, 2001). The initial visits might even be more often, such as once per week, and then reduced. The problem is monitored, and the plan can be changed if it is not effective in controlling the caries. An even more limited goal might be simply a single application of silver diamine fluoride followed by periodic monitoring. In patients with interproximal decay, more frequent bite-wing radiographs can be taken to make monitoring more effective. New diagnostic devices for monitoring caries progression are becoming available but must be used with caution at present as they tend to falsely identify teeth as having decay (Ricketts, 2005).

Strategies With Periodontitis Patients. The gold standard of care for patients with periodontitis remains gingival curettage and frequent scaling and root planing. Such treatment reduces tooth loss associated with periodontitis in adults. However, studies have demonstrated that few patients with periodontal disease will follow professional recommendations for full mouth treatment up to four times per year. For some it is aversive; for others, it is expensive or too time consuming. Many do not truly believe that the treatment is effective. This is true whether the treatment is in a periodontal specialty practice or a general practice. Worse yet, the ability to get patients back is inversely related to the severity of disease. Those with more serious bone loss are less likely to come back than those with less damage.

Rather than try to convince or cajole periodontitis patients into recalls they fail or resent, we offer a compromise. The plan is to help the patient identify those teeth that are critical—for example, abutments of a bridge or removable or anteriors—for chewing or esthetics, and we clean those. We schedule short appointments to anesthetize and thoroughly scale those areas and to irrigate the other pockets with an antimicrobial. Systemic antimicrobials should also be considered. Metronidazole and amoxicillin or ciprofloxin have been used with considerable success. Is this less effective than full mouth scaling? Truly no one knows. What we know is that it is probably more effective than having the patient never return.

What about liability? Isn't this bad care? It is not bad care; it is an alternative. Our clinical experience is that we can slowly increase the number of teeth we are caring for properly over time. Patients who are satisfied with treatment usually become more cooperative and don't disappear. They also become easier to treat.

Shouldn't such patients be sent to the periodontist? The periodontist is a fine alternative if the patient is cooperative. Most periodontitis patients are in fact cared for by dental hygienists in general practices. The general dentist and hygienist have a significant advantage over the specialist because they offer a range of needed services and maintain relationships with patients over long periods of time. Half of our own dental fears patients have serious periodontal bone loss, but few are willing to be referred.

Plan and Implement

Simple strategies such as having open appointment times after school, problem-solving with parents about transportation and timing of appointments, or providing a reduced fee for a series of visits for fluoride varnish or professional toothcleaning can be effective. Remember, the goal is to try to substitute more effective preventive activities for those that are not working.

Dispensing fluorides or high potency fluoride gel toothpastes will likely be more effective than requiring the patient to go the drug store or supermarket. Studies show that mailing fluoridated toothpaste to families is effective in increasing its use and reducing dental caries in children.

Open-ended questions and active listening are the keys to developing an effective strategy. Patients will often agree to a strategy just to get the dental hygienist or preventive assistant off their back. We always find it helpful with both adults and children to get a patient RSVP. That is, we ask the patient whether or not he or she will actually do what we are planning. You'll be surprised how often patients do not intend to follow through and will tell you so if you ask. If that happens, you can problem solve the proposed strategy or choose an alterative.

One clinical approach we have found effective is to ask the patient to try the paste, gel, rinse or varnish in the office. The best example of this is chlorhexidine. Studies show that many patients will reject the chlorhexidine products available in the United States because of bitter taste, tooth sensitivity, or staining. We always ask patients to try the rinse. If a teen spits it out with an "ugh!" there is no sense in dispensing it. If the teen accepts it, you can plan ahead and say that if staining occurs, it can be polished off easily at the next visit. Including strategies such as this in planning with the patient is likely to make the plan more effective.

Monitor and Troubleshoot

Problems can occur almost immediately. The teen's "ugh!" reaction to chlorhexidine is a good example. That is why we almost always try to substitute professional service for home activities, at least initially. As treatment progresses, you make ask patients to keep logs and charts, which are discussed later in this book. You can also take simple steps such as making follow-up phone calls. These calls should be information seeking and problem solving in nature (see the "Motivational Interviewing" chapter). Make the calls positive, and demonstrate that you're taking a special interest in making the strategy work for them. If the patients think you're checking up on them, they will simply tell you what you want to hear—its human nature—and you will not be effective.

Always be ready to adapt and make changes. If coming in before work to get a simple coronal polish and flossing is too difficult for a patient, perhaps it would be better scheduled after work or during lunch hour. If topical fluoride varnish is too yucky, perhaps an alternative fluoride preparation or even toothpaste might be better. If the patient is having trouble finding a flavor of xylitol chewing gum that is acceptable, researching the choices and offering different gums to try at the office will increase your success. Providing a handout with the names and addresses of stores that sell the product will be even more effective.

Remember, the strategies we recommend are designed to increase your batting average. Your success will go up with practice but never to 100 percent. However, employing these strategies will reduce burnout and fatigue in working with patients who find it difficult to follow home care instructions.

"

Asking the right questions takes as much skill
as giving the right answers.

R. Half

As I hear myself talk, I learn what I believe.

D. Bem

"

Chapter 4

Motivating Patients

The Downside of Advice

We want the best for our patients. We want them to lower their risks, engage in healthy behaviors, and choose treatments that lead to optimal health. It is natural for us to try to encourage patients—to give them advice and brochures, even twist their arm gently to get them to cooperate. This challenge is even more difficult when we are working with children. Often we are trying to influence the parent to do or not do something that will affect the child.

When we see a problem, our knee-jerk response as health professionals is to provide advice—an informal version of health education. We have spent much time in classrooms and clinics and would like to share our wisdom with those who will benefit. Giving advice and providing information verbally or through brochures feels good. However, it has a serious downside.

Often patients do not follow our advice. They may not read our brochures, or if they do they quickly forget. Information itself does not change behavior. If it did, we would not have to deal with the sequelae of unhealthy lifestyles—smoking, unwise eating and drinking, etc. Our advice, in fact, may even alienate those we want to help.

We provide advice to people we do not know—to strangers, very often at the initial appointment. We feel compelled; the sooner the person receives the information, the sooner he can change his behavior and benefit. In many clinical settings, the advice giver will never see the recipient again. Advice and information are packaged in a one-time event. There is no relationship, no continuity or follow-up.

This advice-giving approach relies on external motivation. We appeal to the patient or parent by the force of our argument, often with implicit or explicit threats, telling patients and parents what will happen if they do not do what we want them to do right now. We also use the force of our personalities and our status: a person in a white coat who is called "doctor," "dentist," or "therapist" telling an untitled person in street clothing what is best.

An alternate approach relies on identifying or uncovering the internal motivation of the patient or parent. This approach requires two-way communication. We talk and give advice, but we also ask questions and listen. We give the patient or parent choices, and we engage in a discussion of the fit between these choices and the life and lifestyle of the patient or family. This alternate approach requires continuity and follow-up. Small changes are built upon. Continued contact between patient or parent and health provider help support change and allow problem solving.

Motivational Interviewing

This chapter will focus on the alternative approach to advice giving: motivational interviewing (MI). We will provide a brief history of the approach, specify some of its principles and logic, identify skills involved, and spell out the steps required to use this approach in dental settings. Examples will be provided. For readers desiring a more detailed presentation of the motivational interviewing approach in the dental environment, we suggest *Motivate your dental patients: A workbook* (2002) by Phil Weinstein.

History of MI

MI was originally developed for use in alcohol addiction programs in the late 1980s. Shortly afterward the approach was successfully applied to other addictive behaviors, e.g., narcotics use and smoking. Within ten years MI was applied to many other health problems, such as lack of exercise, poor diet, refusal to take medications, unprotected sex, and uncontrolled diabetes. A recent meta-analysis of MI-like approaches was conducted by Burke and his colleagues (2003). Results suggest over a 50 percent improvement rate in decreasing problem drinking and drug use and increasing exercise and proper diet over traditional treatments. Tillis and colleagues (2003) developed a self-report stage-of-change measure to assess commitment to oral self-care (regular interdental cleaning) in more than 700 dental patients. Similarly, Astroth and colleagues (2002) described applications of the stages of change model by dental hygienists. Recently, Weinstein and colleagues (2004) used this approach successfully with the parents of children with a very high risk of caries.

Motivating parents to prevent caries in their young children

(see Weinstein P, Harrison R, Benton T, Motivating parents to prevent caries in their young children, *Journal of the American Dental Association*, 2004 June135:731–8)

OVERVIEW: 240 infants 6–18 months and their parents were randomly assigned to either MI or traditional health education. Parents in the health education condition received a pamphlet and watched a video. Parents in the MI condition also received the pamphlet and watched the video; in addition, they received a personalized MI counseling appointment and six follow-up telephone calls.

ONE-YEAR RESULTS: Children in the MI group had .71 (SD= 2.8) new carious lesions, while those in the health education group had 1.91 (SD= 4.8), a statistically significant difference.

TWO-YEAR RESULTS (see Weinstein P, Harrison R, Benton T, Motivating mothers to prevent caries: Confirming the beneficial effects of counseling, *Journal of the American Dental Association*, 2006 June 137:789–93*)*: Although there was no active intervention during the second year, the differences between groups were maintained.

Stages of Change

According to the Transtheoretical Model of Change, people pass through a process, or stages of change, as they move from accepting the need to change a behavior to maintaining the behavior change. As noted above, most patients do not go to health professionals in a state of readiness to change patterns of behavior that are well established. Here are the stages of change:

Precontemplative: Patients at this stage do not see their behavior as a problem and have no intention of changing. At times they may have tried unsuccessfully to change their behavior. They view the problem as not worth working on, or the probability of success as very small. Patients prefer the status quo to an attempt at change. They are unaware, unable, or unwilling to acknowledge that a problem exists. Movement from this stage to the next should be seen as a major accomplishment in itself.

Contemplative: Patients at this stage are aware a problem exists. They are thinking about making a change, about acting. Yet they are unsure and "ambivalent" about making a change. While they think about the benefits ("pros"), they also focus on the costs or negatives ("cons") associated with the change. Almost every potential change has potential problems. These patients are not yet committed to action, yet they are uncomfortable with the status quo.

Preparation/action: Patients at this third stage are ready to change and have made personal commitments. They see the benefits as outweighing the costs of change. A plan is developed and implemented.

Maintenance: This stage follows once the behavior change has been maintained for at least six months. Just as maintaining abstinence from substance abuse is crucial, maintaining positive health behaviors is extremely important. However, these positive behaviors tend to deteriorate over time (usually from six months to a year). This deterioration often results in termination of the new and positive change and often to a relapse into an earlier stage of change. Awareness of potential relapses and what to do about them are important. More important than the lapse itself is the discouragement associated with it.

The Stages of Change perspective has been useful in providing a framework for understanding how individuals change a wide range of problem behaviors, from smoking to overeating. The importance of this model lies in the fact that strategies and activities to promote change differ significantly across stages. Individuals in different stages utilize different processes of change; processes vary with stages. Establishing the stage in which a person "resides" and deciding upon the course of treatment based on that stage promotes individualization of treatment.

How Does MI Work?

The MI approach helps people move through stages of change, from being in denial that a problem exists to maintaining new health-related behaviors over time. MI counseling provides support for the patient; it is non-judgmental, non-confrontational, and tries to be patient-centered.

The MI approach is patient and recognizes that not everyone is ready to change what they are doing at a given point in time. Readiness is a continuum. Movement along the continuum, from being unaware or being in denial to being willing to think about change, is an acceptable short-term outcome. There will be other opportunities.

> SUCCESSFUL COUNSELORS GET PATIENTS TO TALK;
> UNSUCESSFUL COUNSELORS DO ALL OF THE TALKING.

Patients are encouraged to talk as much as or more than those doing the counseling. In fact, research on this technique actually compares the amount of patient talk to health professional talk. Results suggest the more patients talk, the better.

To help understand MI, it is useful to point out its roots. Let's briefly go over the two components—client-centered psychotherapy and behavior change technology.

Client-Centered Psychotherapy

Client-centered psychotherapy encourages the counselor or therapist to establish a "therapeutic alliance" (a close working relationship with a patient). Without such an alliance nothing of value can be accomplished or maintained. By forming such an alliance, counselors establish rapport and win and maintain the trust of their clients and patients.

To begin with, the counselor must be warm and genuine, that is, must be approachable and be really concerned about the welfare of the patient or client. Empathy with the patient and client is stressed. When the client believes the counselor is empathic—that is, when he or she believes the counselor understands her/him and the problems—it is only then that movement toward the solution of problems can occur.

Empathy is established when the counselor asks open-ended questions and then demonstrates listening skills. Empathy is built when the patient knows we care enough to ask questions and take the time to demonstrate that we are listening.

Proper posture and eye contact are very helpful in letting a person know we are listening. What we say is critical. The key is reflecting what the person is saying by summarizing and paraphrasing.

"Resistance" is an old psychotherapeutic concept. The concept is evoked when the patient, who seeks out help, does not change, often in a situation where he is clearly hurting and in turmoil. In health care settings we have found that patients often resist advice, especially unsolicited advice. The more we try to justify the advice, the more the resistance, usually in the form of disagreeing with the advice, its benefit, or its practicality. Such conflicts, even when the advice is to benefit the patient or child, engender reactance, the tendency to assert one's independence when personal freedom is threatened (by being told what to do).

Think of the teen who is ordered to pick up his room, or throw out the trash right now!

Client-centered psychotherapy is sensitive to this problem. Counselors are trained to be sensitive to advice-giving traps that lead to reactance. They stress that the client is in charge, is responsible, and makes the decisions. Although there is no overt persuasion, the counselor steers the discussion by asking the right questions and by reflecting, amplifying, and helping interpret thoughts and feelings. The approach is subtle; although indirect, it is not without goals.

HOW DOES SOMEONE KNOW YOU REALLY CARE?
ASK MEANINGFUL QUESTIONS.
DEMONSTRATE THAT YOU LISTEN TO THE ANSWER.

Behavior change technology

In client-centered psychotherapy, the client not only identifies the problem but also identifies the solution. The counselor does not suggest solutions. Using the behavior change paradigm, the MI counselor suggests solutions, engages with the client or patient in problem solving, strengthens the person's resolve to change, and provides suggestions on HOW to implement and maintain the change over time. Overall, the MI counselor provides direction but does not provide advice prematurely—that is, before there is a relationship, before there is trust.

Client-centered psychotherapy and behavior change are melded together. In MI, the former is used to establish a therapeutic alliance and to help the patient identify the problem. The latter is used to identify and implement solutions.

How long does MI take?

MI and its offshoot counseling strategies used in health settings, such as dental clinics, are brief. The initial counseling in a dental setting requires a minimum of 3-15 minutes and, depending on the problem and the individual, can benefit from more time. Short follow-up discussions, in person or on the phone, are part of the counseling.

MI is similar to horse whispering. In MI and horse whispering, trust and the building of an alliance are essential. The client and the horse interact and are led gently down a mutually defined path.

MI Skills

The effectiveness of MI depends on the skill of the practitioner. The MI approach will increase the success rate of most practitioners. Those who practice and develop basic MI skills will have the highest rates of success. MI skills include asking open-ended questions, reflective listening, and encouraging self-efficacy. Knowledge of behavioral technology and practice in using the technology in a clinical setting are also very helpful and will be reviewed later in this book.

Asking open-ended questions

Asking open-ended questions is not difficult. An open-ended question cannot be answered by a yes or a no; it encourages the patient to express him or herself. Asking yes-no questions, especially at the beginning of an appointment, teaches the patient to give short, simple answers, rather than the sort of elaboration needed for MI counseling. Moreover, asking "yes" or "no" questions implies that the interaction is taking place between an active professional and a passive patient.

Close-ended questions are usually phrased with words such as, "Do you?" "Are you?" "Have you?" "Will you?" "Can you?" These questions are useful only when little detail is required and factual information is being verified. Open-ended questions are usually phrased with words such as, "Tell me," or "Describe," "How?" "What?" "Which?"

SAY: "Tell me about your dental problems."

DO NOT SAY: "Do you have any dental problems?"

Try not to ask too many open-ended questions in a row; three is about the limit. Open-ended questions give us the opportunity to use reflective listening.

Reflective listening

Reflective listening is a response to what is said that shows your understanding. What is said often can be ambiguous or have multiple meanings. Reflective listening is a way of checking to be sure of the meaning. Only people who are really concerned and interested in the person and her situation try to be sure.

Reflective listening is one of the most essential and most challenging skills to be mastered in the MI approach. A dental health professional who cannot listen reflectively cannot use MI counseling. Many of us believe we have these skills, but we are usually rusty. It takes considerable practice. It is not enough to read this book and to do an exercise or two.

Most of us associate listening with being passive, perhaps bored. People prefer the role of the talker to that of the listener. We are focused on our own ideas and points of view. When we are thinking about what to say next, we may not be listening.

Listening is considered an expression of empathy. We want our patients to see us as interested in their lives and their dental problems. Listening also encourages patients to talk. Patient talking is the key to helping the patient act or change, as what we say is what we believe, not the other way around.

Trying to convince others to change or act usually does not work; it leads them to talk about why they cannot change or act (and they are the experts on their lives). Hearing themselves say they cannot act is deadly. When patients are ambivalent, desiring to act or change but unsure they can, the MI counseling approach suggests reflecting the feeling of ambivalence, discussing the value of the act or change, and problem solving.

When listening, try not to interrupt, ask additional questions, or give advice. The interviewer must appear non-judgmental. Nonverbal cues are also important. Lean forward slightly, nod your head when appropriate, and maintain eye contact if the patient is North American or European. Please see the chapter on "Communicating With Your Patients" for more discussion of culturally-appropriate communication styles.

When using reflective listening, the interviewer attempts to feed back to the person the essence of what she has just said. This is done by paraphrasing or summarizing and responds not only to what the patient said but to her feelings.

There is more than one type of reflective listening. The following three types should be used after you have practiced them.

Simple reflection. Use the patient's words and your words to paraphrase. Summarize briefly at intervals to keep the conversation going or to help transition to another topic.

Patient: "I have always really hated the way my front teeth look. My parents did not have the resources to deal with the problem. Now I want to do something about it."

Dental professional: "The way your teeth look has bothered you for a long time. It sounds like you are ready to work on that problem."

Amplified reflection This is similar to simple reflection, but with enthusiasm.

Dental professional: "It sounds like you are REALLY ready to work on this problem that has been bothering you for a long time."

Double-sided reflection This reflects ambivalence that has been revealed by the patient.

"On the one hand you feel (think).... On the other..."

When you believe a patient is ambivalent, reflect both pros and cons. This allows discussion of both. We can elicit motivational self-statements and problem solve to overcome the cons. Double-sided reflection also presents the appearance of being fair and evenhanded.

Dental professional: "You seem to be telling me that you really want to get that gap between your front teeth fixed, but you are concerned that others will notice a big change and that you will be embarrassed. Did I get it right?"

Exercises

The following exercises involve groups of three. Each learner will practice and receive feedback. If time permits, play all three persons: speaker, listener, and observer. The following form is useful in providing feedback:

OBSERVER CHECKLIST

____ Uses open-ended questions

How many? ______________________________

____ Uses reflective listening

____ Simple reflections

____ Amplified reflections

____ Double-sided reflections

____ Gives advice, suggestions

____ Reassures

____ Interrupts, asks questions, changes topic

____ Judgmental expression

Comments:____

First exercise:

Person 1 will tell person 2 about a vacation, trip, birthday, or dinner plan that did not work out.

Person 1 will reveal the information reluctantly and slowly.

Person 2 will use as many reflective listening techniques as possible.

Person 3 will give feedback to Person 2. Person 1 will also comment on the interview.

Second exercise:

Person 1 is a new patient who has had a bad dental experience at a previous office or clinic.

Person 2 will try to establish rapport and trust and then ask about previous dental experiences.

Person 3 will give feedback to Person 2. Person 1 will also comment on the interview.

Third exercise:

Person 1 is himself or herself

Person 2 asks, "Tell me about what you would like to change in yourself."

Person 3 again provides feedback.

Encouraging self-efficacy

The concept of self-efficacy refers to an individual's belief in her ability to carry out or succeed in a specific task or action. When self-efficacy is high, the patient believes the change or act is feasible, and she tries and persists. When self-efficacy is low, she believes she will not be successful, leading to resistant comments and a lack of effort.

A metaphor is useful here. If you do not believe you can win the lottery you will not buy a ticket. However, you cannot win without that ticket. Essentially, we recognize it takes confidence to proceed in specific ways. Low general confidence may be a characteristic of the patient; however, she may be led to believe that it is within her abilities to make a specific action or change. This belief mediates the attempt.

The overall message we are conveying is: "You can do it! You can be successful, just try it." This approach is especially useful when we encourage small steps. "Don't change how you clean your whole mouth; for now, just focus on this spot, right here." Here we function as coaches, helping patients by encouraging steps toward do-able goals.

Social support and affirmations

Social support enhances self-efficacy. It is usually provided verbally and can take many forms. Basically, providing social support involves lots of positive comments. The following are examples:

I appreciate how hard it is for you… you took a big step coming here.

I know you really want to… I think it's great. I hope you are proud of yourself.

I am not sure about how you think about it, but from what you have told me I really believe you will be able to…

Wow, you seem like you are going to go ahead and try to get that great smile you told me you wanted. Good for you!

You have just said that making these changes will not be easy, but you seem very dedicated to finding a way to save your teeth. That is incredible.

Self-motivational statements

Try to elicit self-motivational statements in all interactions with your patients. This involves cuing them to tell you about the problem, their concern and intention to change, or their optimism in the process of acting or changing. This encourages self-efficacy. The following are examples:

Tell me what encourages you.

Tell me about the advantages of going ahead now. Why is this a good time?

You seem to be optimistic. Tell me what you are thinking.

Tell me about how you see the disadvantages (if you believe the patient is not ready to change or act) and the advantages of the approach we are talking about.

As this example indicates, it may be useful to ask about the cons as a preface to asking about the positive aspects of change.

Every self-motivational statement by the patient is capable of minimizing resistance and tipping the balance a bit farther toward change or action. If a statement comes from the patient's own mouth, it has validity for him

Additional strategies

The more we know about a patient, the more ammunition we have to encourage him. Uncovering pride in business, job, school, sports, and hobbies allows you to point to competencies that can transfer to the problem at hand.

Telling success stories of previous patients with similar problems can be helpful. Such stories function as metaphors—if they can do it, you can do it.

Step-by-step MI

Here is a detailed description of the steps MI counselors follow, usually in sequence:

Step 1: Establish Rapport and Trust.

Establishing a therapeutic alliance between health care professional and patient is necessary for change. In recent years the importance of this bond has been repeatedly demonstrated in all the helping professions. Rapport and trust are required for this alliance to flourish. Here are some of the many strategies to establish rapport and trust:

> Advice from a stranger falls on deaf ears.
>
> **Don't be a stranger to your patient!**

Rapport-building strategies:

1. Share mutual interests, briefly.
   "Tell me about what you like to do when you have the time." Such a request allows you to comment, briefly, on mutual interests, and even to request a small favor that demonstrates interest, such as, "Can you give me the name and address of that shop, campground, web site, etc.?"
2. Demonstrate concern by asking important, open-ended questions, and then listening.
   "How are your teeth treating you?"

"What do you want from your teeth?"
"What is it like to have... (describe the dental problems)? How does it affect your life?"
"What is it like to be Duane's mom (Duane being a hyperactive six year old), etc.?"

3. Provide positive, caring comments (affirmations).
"The drive here was long and hard; you must really want to feel/look better."
"You seem to be very concerned/dedicated to your child's welfare; you are a caring, loving mom."
"I love your child's outfit. Where did you find matching..."?
"I can see you are a very well-organized and competent person."
4. Play or interact briefly with the child in the waiting room or operatory. Playing and interacting with a child demonstrates to many parents that you are approachable and like children.
5. Provide continuity. Let the patients know you will personally see and/or talk to them again. Let them know at the beginning of the initial appointment.

Trust-building strategies

Many people feel dental and medical personnel are judgmental and do not understand what it is like to walk a mile in their shoes. They may report that in the past they have not had real choice or information about treatment or may not have had the opportunity to influence how the treatment was delivered. Some do not believe that dental or medical personnel put the patient's interest first; such people feel taken advantage of, cheated, or disrespected.

Distrustful people may feel victimized, trapped by higher-status dental personnel, and unable to assert their feelings to people dressed in white and surgical gowns. Some may seem resentful and angry—even when they are new patients in your office or clinic!

Building trust involves enhancing one's sense of personal control. The following strategies are useful:

1. Encourage the patient to tell you his story (what happened in the

past). Listen and be sure to let him know you understand what happened. This is very reassuring.

2. Ask the distrustful patient whether or not she wants information and what sort of information is best. Distrustful patients not only want to know what will happen and what the procedure will feel like, but want to understand the rationale or the science behind the procedure. Detailed explanations are often very important for periodontal maintenance patients, who are exposed to costly, invasive procedures that may be confused with routine coronal prophylaxis. This is the patient to whom you can show off what you have learned in your recent Continuing Dental Education (CDE) course and study club. This patient will love to look at radiographs with you as you explain about her disease and what the treatment entails.
3. Distrustful patients like to watch procedures. Offer the patient a mirror and explain what is going on, perhaps as a running technical commentary.
4. Distrustful patients like written treatment plans, treatment options, and the opportunity to discuss the plans with someone they trust. This is not the patient you pressure to choose the option you desire in a timely manner or face dire consequences, e.g., tooth loss, pain, embarrassment, etc. A high-pressure approach is known to backfire with those who are distrustful.
5. This is the patient for whom you invite another set of eyes and ears (patient's spouse, trusted friend, or relative) to the consultation.
6. This is also the patient to whom you suggest a second opinion. Such a suggestion is reassuring to a distrustful patient, as only a competent, honest person would make such a suggestion.

Step 2: Ask questions and help the patient make an argument for change

It is useful to let the patient talk and hear himself voice the need to change. This helps him identify the problem that will motivate change.

We are helpers; the patient is responsible for the decision to act or change. He will consider acting or changing when he perceives he has a problem.

We help patients identify problems by asking meaningful questions (and by listening to the answers). Technically, according to MI literature, we are helping to create a discrepancy between present behavior and important personal goals. Patient statements that reveals these goals, which they may not have been aware of themselves or perhaps have even denied to others, are called self-motivational statements. MI counseling tries to prompt patients to make such statements repeatedly.

Step 2 involves movement from the first stage (Precontemplative) to the second stage (Contemplative).

Here are some examples of meaningful questions:

"Tell me about your teeth and the teeth of your older child (who has stainless steel crowns). What do you want for your baby?

"Suppose you were granted a 'dental miracle,' (or an 'extreme makeover'). What would happen?"

"If you do not do anything, what will happen?"

"What would you do (for your dental health, appearance, etc.), if you could?"

"Tell me how you feel about your teeth."

"How can we make things better?"

Other ideas?

Write them here:

Patients may not hear you when you recommend change; it is far more powerful for patients to hear themselves say they have a problem.

WHAT WE SAY IS WHAT WE BELIEVE, NOT THE OTHER WAY AROUND

Here are a few more open-ended questions to which a person must use his own words to respond.

"Tell me some good things and some not so good things about your teeth."

"Was there ever a time you did not have dental problems? What was it like? What do you want, if it were possible, for the future?"

Step 3: Encourage self-motivational statements

After asking questions, listen for self-motivational statements and reflect them back to the patient or parent. This includes patients in the Contemplative stage. Step 3 occurs with Step 2 early in the MI process, and it does not stop. Counselors continue to try to elicit self-motivational statements through all stages of change.

Dental professional: "Tell me about YOUR teeth and the teeth of your family?"

Patient: "We have bad teeth that have caused us much misery and embarrassment over the years."

Dental professional: "Your teeth have caused suffering."

Patient: "Yes, just last week … I've got to do something with my teeth."

Dental professional: "You are telling me you are ready to move forward with dental treatment to end your suffering. Did I get it right?"

If the patient is ambivalent, reflect the ambivalence with a double-sided or amplified reflection.

Patient: "I really want to have my teeth look (feel) better. I have a few concerns, but I think I can do this, now that I am here."

Dental professional: "(Wow!) You are telling me, all things considered, you think you will be successful. Great!"

The previous examples focus on recognition of self-motivational statements. Here are some questions you can ask questions to elicit them.

"Remind me why you are doing this."

"What makes you think you need to do something?"

"What would be the advantage of stopping smoking?"

"What makes you think, if you decide to go ahead, you will be successful?"

The more the patient or parent talks about the problem, her intent to act or change, and her optimism, the better. Acknowledging a problem and voicing determination to solve it facilitates action.

> After the patient or parent makes a self-motivational statement, provide reinforcement and encouragement. Ask:
> "On a scale of 1-10, where 10 is as much as I have ever wanted anything and 1 is just a little, how much do you want to...?"
> "Oh great! A four! Wow, you really do want your teeth to be more attractive.
> What would happen if you do nothing?"
> Respond with enthusiasm, even if the patient or parent indicates lukewarm desire.

Step 4: Helping prepare for change

When the patient or parent begins to make self-motivational statements, he or she is contemplating action and the problems or difficulties associated with it. Although it is useful to continue to encourage self-motivational statements, the MI counselor now identifies the "cons" (obstacles or hurdles that interfere with action) and encourages a plan that will minimize or overcome these interferences.

When the counselor believes the patient is very aware of the problem and desires to change or act, she begins to provide additional direction. She asks permission to problem solve with the patient or parent.

Examples:

"You have given me reasons why you want to.... May I share some ideas with you that have worked for other patients?"

"Would you like to hear what has worked for other moms in this community?"

Once permission is provided, give the patient choices. If you work in a setting in which the same problem reappears very often, you may want to provide the patient with a written "menu" of options that others have successfully used.

The following boxed example is the actual menu we used with the mothers of toddlers 6-18 months old who were at high risk for early childhood caries:

> **Menu**
>
> - ❑ Do not let anyone add anything sugary to your child's bottle.
> - ❑ Clean baby's teeth daily as soon as they appear.
> - ❑ Use a very small amount of fluoride toothpaste.
> - ❑ Hold your baby when feeding, then lay the baby down to sleep; if the baby wakens give water, not milk or juice.
> - ❑ Use a cup.
> - ❑ Offer snacks no more than 2-3 times a day.
> - ❑ Remind the hygienist or assistant to paint the baby's teeth with protective fluoride.

After we present the menu to the parents, we go over each item briefly. We discuss the items that they are interested in a second time, more thoroughly. We ask the parents to brainstorm other ideas not on the menu. We caution them not to try to implement all of the items. We focus on a subset that is do-able and discuss the problems they will have in going ahead.

When parents or patients ask us what we would do, we respond that they are the experts on their life. Therefore they are responsible, not us. Our job is to point out and help discuss options and to provide support.

> Don't forget to discuss the issues (cons) that will interfere with action. Emphasize patient choice; caries and periodontal disease are multi-factorial problems with many possible solutions. These problems are chronic, not acute. We do not

> have to have an optimal solution in place immediately. We have time to phase in or try out various solutions. A huge dental treatment plan that overwhelms the patient has little likelihood of success. A plan that phases in various treatments over time is preferable.

During this step we avoid one-sided discussions that focus only on benefits. Such conversations appear coercive. We help identify the problems patients will have in implementation. We help discriminate what the patient or parents can readily do from actions that will probably be more difficult. We recommend that low-hanging fruit be picked first. Make it easy to be successful. Remember you can recommend additional actions in subsequent sessions. If we overwhelm the patient, we decrease the probability that he will continue to work on the problem.

The goal of this step in the MI process is to develop a plan for change. The plans that work best are in writing. We give patients a copy of the menu with the actions that they have agreed to do ticked off in red. A photocopy goes into the chart. We encourage the patient to make the plan public. Telling others what we will do increases the likelihood of action.

Although a menu is useful, it is not necessary. Some counselors tell success stories of clients they have helped and explore the possibility that what worked for others may work for the present client. Some even show before-and-after photos. Once a plan has been developed, we ask that the patient try it out. We suggest an "experiment." For example, patients are more likely to try out new tooth-cleaning behaviors as an experiment than if they are making long-term commitments.

When we are helping patients form plans, we put in as many details as possible. We help patients think about the circumstances in their lives that can help or hinder the development of habits. We ask, to continue the above example, if remembering to engage in the new tooth cleaning behavior may be a problem. If remembering will be a problem, we suggest strategies to cue the new behavior. We often suggest the use of the Premack Principle. (See the "Planning an Intervention" chapter.)

Warning: It is too easy to overestimate a patient's readiness. That is, we frequently believe the patient is ready to act when she has not decided. She may be merely verbalizing what she believes should be said in response to the social pressures of the situation. Slow down. Be sure the patient has thought about the cons and is willing to proceed.

Step 5: Responding to resistance

Resistance is normal; it should be expected. Resistance should be looked at as the flip side of motivation. Minimize resistance, maximize motivation; allow resistance to blossom, motivation dissipates.

There are various forms of resistance, active and passive. Arguing, interrupting, denying, minimizing the problem, being pessimistic or fatalistic, and ignoring or sidetracking the discussion are typical.

What should you do when you are aware the patient is demonstrating resistance? Psychology literature provides us with insight into resistance and strategies to use. Here are some guidelines:

1. **Think of resistance as a signal, a red light to stop and do something different.** This is the most important guideline. Most of the time patients show resistance when you are moving too fast and/or do not understand them and the situation. A patient may not be in the stage you believe him to be or may be ambivalent.
2. **Avoid arguing or debating.** Defending your point of view only leads to more defensiveness. The force of your argument will not alter resistance, only perhaps its form. Patients who argue and hear themselves telling you why they cannot act or change will not act or change.
3. **Drop the expert role.** Avoid being authoritative. You have probably been talking too much. Ask an open-ended question and use reflective listening.
4. **Emphasize choice and encourage an active patient role.** Tell the patient, "I'm not here to make decisions for you; it's truly your choice." Encourage self-motivational comments. "Tell me again

what you want to happen." "What happens if you do nothing?" Encourage discussion and problem solving.

5. **Involve family members when possible.** Identify family (or friends) who may be concerned about the problem. Are those people supportive? If so, ask the patient to include them in creating and implementing a plan.
6. **Agree with the patient; side with the negative.** This is not the first strategy we would use; however, it can be effective. Agree with the patient in a way that demonstrates empathy, not disdain. Acknowledge the difficulties, the truth as the patient sees it. Interestingly, when you agree, the patient often argues for the action or change! The following are examples:

   "Coming in for deep scaling four times a year presents too many problems.... But they are only teeth. Right?"

   "I know you really are concerned about the health of your children, but your child may grow up and have serious dental problems, like you do, even though you hope otherwise..."

   "You are telling me it seems too hard....You cannot see yourself doing this."

Step 6: Responding to provoking comments

Patients often have beliefs that keep them from acting or changing. These beliefs often reflect folk mores, family history, or conventional wisdom that is out-of-date. What we say when a patient or parent makes one of these comments may determine the outcome of our counseling.

You may have heard some people say, "My family has always had dental problems; we have bad genes... soft teeth." What do you say to such provoking comments?

Although the natural response is to provide corrective information, the information often will be interpreted as criticism, a denial of a patient's beliefs and experiences. The corrective information is likely to result in a counter-argument or in the patient "rolling over." Rolling

> **FATALISM AND DENIAL**
>
> Some patients believe tooth loss is inevitable and that dental treatment is ineffective in controlling tooth attrition. For these people, dental treatment is for emergencies only. They and their parents often have not experienced the benefits of regular dental care. These people are often fatalistic, denying that anything but temporary pain control is possible. Given this logic, extractions are the only rational solution.

over is the patient's decision to superficially acquiesce. It is the "yes, doctor" response to an authority that actually means "no."

Agreeing with the patient is useful. For example:

Patient: "My family has always had huge dental problems. We all have soft teeth..."

Dental professional: "There is definitely a genetic component to dental problems. A few years ago we used to think there was nothing we could do to help people with this problem. But research has given us some solutions. Are you interested in hearing what we can do for people with soft teeth?"

Patient: "Well, I guess so."

Here we agree with the patient. We are agreeing that the patient is vulnerable to dental disease. Our recommendation will reflect the genetic high risk. We are communicating in a way that the patient can understand.

Let's try another.

Dental professional: "We are interested in protecting your child's teeth so he will not have cavities."

Parent: "But they are only baby teeth."

Dental professional: "I know. Dentists used to think baby teeth were not important, but we have learned a few things recently. If there is an infection in the baby teeth, there will be an infection in the permanent teeth for the rest of the person's life.... Early loss of baby teeth also can result in crooked teeth..."

Again, we agree with the patient and communicate new information—the importance of baby teeth.

Step 7: Follow-up and relapse

Before you say good-bye to the patient, be sure she understands that you will be available for follow-up. Anticipate problems. Tell her you expect there will be bumps in the road. You can discuss possible problems and solutions. For example, what will she say to a grandmother who wants to put sugar in the baby's bottle? Remind her that plans may need to be adjusted. Tell the patient to feel free to contact you to problem-solve.

Toward that end, schedule brief follow-up telephone contacts or actual visits. Try to arrange to call a patient at within a given time window. ("What is the best time to call you?") Call or visit after two weeks, then a month. Frequent follow-up is very helpful and is not time consuming. Postcard reminders can also be used.

Relapse of new self-care behaviors is normal. See other chapters in this book for discussion of relapse and relapse prevention.

Assignment for Chapter 4

For your first assignment, we suggest that you identify in writing three problems you, a patient, or an acquaintance are probably willing to own. Remember, you need not try to manufacture hypothetical problems. We all have real problems and know people with real problems worth working on. Some examples of projects with which other practitioners have had success include: increasing brushing, flossing, or toothpicking; ceasing or reducing smoking or alcohol consumption; increasing headgear compliance; losing weight or making diet and nutritional changes, especially reduction of cariogenic food intake; beginning and carrying out regular exercise programs, such as the aerobics program recommended by Cooper (1970); cessation of nailbiting or thumbsucking; increasing study time; decreasing patient anxiety to manageable levels; increasing or decreasing wearing of dentures or night guard; decreasing child misbehavior in the operatory.

Problem #1

1. Whose problem is it (patient, spouse, friend, self)?
2. What stage of change is the person currently in? How do you know this?
3. What would you say or do to help move the person to the next stage of change?
4. Describe the problem.

Problem #2

1. Whose problem is it (patient, spouse, friend, self)?
2. What stage of change is the person currently in? How do you know this?
3. What would you say or do to help move the person to the next stage of change?
4. Describe the problem.

Problem #3

1. Whose problem is it (patient, spouse, friend, self)?
2. What stage of change is the person currently in? How do you know this?
3. What would you say or do to help move the person to the next stage of change?
4. Describe the problem.

Teachers are costly, but bad teachers cost more.

B. Talbert

Where there is the necessary technical skill to move mountains, there is no need for the faith that moves mountains.

D. Bem

Chapter 5

Teaching Skills

Plaque control is crucial to prevention and control of gingivitis, periodontitis, and dental caries. Learning to provide effective personal hygiene training is very important for any clinician. When patients effectively remove plaque, whether with a toothbrush or with a chemical agent such as 0.12% chlorhexidine mouth rinse, no gingivitis or caries develops (Loe *et al.*, 1972). Inflamed gingival tissues heal rapidly when plaque is removed via daily oral hygiene (Loe *et al.*, 1965). On the other hand, inflammation takes several days to develop if a tooth is not cleaned at all. Meticulous oral hygiene at intervals of 48 hours generally results in a healthy mouth (Lang *et al.*, 1973). This conclusion makes sense because the initial colonizers of tooth surfaces are harmless microflora. Only later, if the conditions are right, do pathogenic microorganisms infiltrate the plaque biofilm. In the absence of oral hygiene and with frequent sugar intake, incipient dental caries will develop by two weeks.

What should we do when a patient is unable, even if his life depended on it, to effectively use a toothbrush or interdental cleaning aid?

If the person has a skill deficiency, how do you teach the desired behavior in the first place? Sometimes all the encouragement or reinforcement in the world will not enable the patient to skillfully use an interdental brush. The problem is that first you must produce the behavior so that you can encourage it to continue. To begin, we will focus on the techniques that can be used to establish new behavior patterns. Most clinicians are familiar with many of these techniques, as they are part of the health-education model of prevention. The techniques are effective if the problem is a lack of knowledge or skill.

Introducing Skills

How you introduce skill training to patients is extremely important. We recognize most patients are already involved in some sort of regular oral self-care activity. Unfortunately, their home care is not usually effective in fully removing plaque. Patients do not see what they are doing. They often miss problem areas or give them only brief and superficial cleaning.

Most of us believe that we learned how to brush our teeth adequately at an early age. In fact, some patients are insulted when told they need to learn better home-care skills. Consequently, how this topic is introduced is important. We suggest a low-key approach. For example: "Would you like to learn some tips about how to brush more effectively?" Or, "Research has just uncovered new facts about brushing and flossing. Would you like to hear about them?" "Could I have your permission to show you how to take less time with your cleaning but be more effective?" The general approach we have found most effective is to liken self-care to an athletic skill. Imagine the following conversation:

Patient: "Boy, the L.A. Lakers are sure going to town." Or, "Sure glad the weather is getting better, I can't wait to start playing tennis again."

Dental Hygienist: "I know what you mean. I think of the ability to clean teeth as very similar to any athletic skill. It takes practice and real concentration to perform well. Are you interested in improving your dental game?"

Patient: "Well, if I don't have to work too hard."

Dental Hygienist: "Fortunately, you don't have to practice four hours a day to be an expert at cleaning your teeth! Let me see how you do now and I'll give you some pointers on how to improve your skills."

The patient is under great social pressure not only to tell you that he cleans his teeth and gums regularly at home, but also to show you how proficient he is. We capitalize on this tendency by encouraging him to do the best job possible as we send him to the sink to demonstrate. From watching, we learn whether the patient is capable of optimal cleaning skills. We also learn how long it takes. Obviously, the longer he takes, the less likely it is that he will duplicate that effort at home; thus, our efforts may focus on improving his efficiency. We apply disclosing solution. If the patient sits back down after cleaning and the disclosing solution reveals significant plaque, especially in high risk or vulnerable areas, we must first concentrate on teaching the basics of plaque removal.

Patient demonstrations of cleaning often reveal serious deficiencies in skill. Kleber *et al.* (1981) and MacGreggor and Rugg-Gunn (1979) have indicated that lingual surfaces are the areas most commonly omitted by children during toothbrushing. The Kleber study showed that more than 80 percent of the children in each group, from baseline to the end of the study, failed to brush the right and left lingual surfaces of the mandibular or maxillary dentition. Overall, 38 percent of the dental surfaces were not brushed. Similarly MacGreggor and Rugg-Gunn observed that the anterior labial surfaces were brushed most often and the lingual surfaces least often.

Findings for adults are similar. Robinson (1946) found that toothbrushing was almost entirely confined to buccal and labial surfaces. More recently, Cumming and Loe (1973) found that buccal and labial surfaces had less plaque than lingual surfaces. Dexterity, even in adults, may be a factor. Kenney *et al.* (1976) determined that manual dexterity of the right or preferred hand showed significant correlation with oral hygiene scores. Right-handed patients do better cleaning the left side of the mouth.

In teaching oral hygiene, it is easy to give the patient the impression that oral disease occurs equally throughout the oral cavity. Epidemiologists have shown that periodontal disease and caries are not uniformly distributed in the mouth, and that the surfaces and gum tissues affected change with age. Tooth decay in children is most likely on the occlusal surfaces; in adults, the interproximal surfaces are involved, especially where there are already fillings. In children, rapidly progressive juvenile periodontitis strikes the primary molars and incisors; in adults, periodontal destruction takes a different distribution. Root surface caries is a major problem in older persons, especially in the mandibular molars.

On the other hand, in toothbrushing populations, most of the unremoved dental plaque is interproximal. Thus, we need eventually to introduce interdental cleaning, but not initially.

As clinicians, few of us take a long-term perspective. Generally, the rate of disease progression, especially for gingivitis and early periodontal disease, or even for caries in a fluoridated area, is not so fast that everything must be accomplished in one session. Thus, it may be better to focus on one problem per teaching session. If the patient will be in the practice for 30 years, there will be many opportunities for instruction. In fact, we find that patients avoid practices that are too aggressive in "changing" them. If you find through assessment and observation that the patient is ineffective with a toothbrush, then target this skill as the primary concern. Better yet, focus on a particular quadrant or sextant. Do not introduce more skills (e.g., flossing or toothpicking) at this time. Our clinical studies of private practices have revealed that too often the patient is overwhelmed with dental cleaning devices when what is needed is improvement in fundamental toothbrushing skill. Here is the recommended strategy:

- Observe the patient's current skill level (often using disclosing solutions).
- Devise a plan for modification, demonstrating your approach.
- Have the patient practice under supervision.

Our studies show that the average instructional session in private practice lasts less than 10 minutes; this, amount of instruction is plenty for one lesson with limited goals.

New patients in early stages of periodontal or restorative treatment may need a number of short sessions to bring existing skills to an effective level. In our own practice, this is the task of the dental hygienist or dental assistant. Initial therapy for periodontal conditions often lasts four to five visits as we perform the treatment under local anesthesia by quadrants. At each session we use five minutes for instruction. Taking up a whole appointment for instruction is less effective for us because the patient ends up getting too much information and too many tools to clean with. Further, the fee we receive for periodontal therapy more than covers the cost of short instructional lessons.

Teaching the Patient New Skills

Some form of modeling helps when patients attempt a first approximation of the behavior. You may have seen children play a game called "monkey see, monkey do," where one youngster does something, like raising his hands over his head, and the other children imitate him. This game illustrates modeling, one of the most basic and effective ways to learn new behavior (Bandura, 1969).

Have you ever tried to learn how to do something by reading about how to do it or having someone tell you? You may have had difficulty. Contrast this situation with one in which someone demonstrates or models the behavior. For example, you are using modeling when you teach a patient how to brush properly by demonstrating on a plastic model or on your own teeth.

You should not expect a new, complex behavior to emerge full-blown or spontaneously after the first try. Similarly, once your patients know how to perform the behavior in question, it is perhaps too much to ask that they suddenly start to perform it consistently and religiously.

Another valuable technique is suggesting that a patient begin cleaning at the same point in the mouth each time and go slowly through the mouth systematically. It does not matter where the patient begins except that common sense suggests (1) brushing the most important teeth—molars and premolars—first, and (2) keeping the brush on one area, even one tooth, for long enough to clean. We find that having the patient put the brush on a particular spot and clean, counting to 4 or 5 slowly, is helpful. Don't let the patient proceed to the next tooth surface until the first one is clean. Slowing patients down and having them actually look at what they are cleaning is very effective.

It is beyond the scope of this text to provide a technical discussion of the myriad oral hygiene implements available to the conscientious practitioner today. The interested reader is referred to two fine texts: *Primary Preventive Dentistry* by Harris and Garcia-Godoy (Prentice Hall, 2004) and *Preventive Materials, Methods, and Programs* by Axelsson (Quintessence Books, 2004). They contain chapters on toothbrushes, auxiliary tooth cleaning aids, dentifrices, rinses, and oral irrigation.

The Toothbrush Is Underutilized

In most practices we have observed, the toothbrush is underutilized, and other aids, especially dental floss, are introduced too early and with little real understanding of how difficult they are to use. In our practice, we do not expect a patient to learn brushing and flossing at the same time. If a patient does not brush efficaciously, we do not introduce further implements until the problem is remedied.

We emphasize flexibility. Most patients believe they must brush three times a day to be healthy. Where did they learn this? From us, of course! However, by simplifying the task—say, to brush well once a day—we reduce its difficulty. Emphasize that the *quality*, not the *quantity*, of cleaning is most important in oral health.

Exhaustive studies on various types of toothbrushes fail to show any meaningful differences between types of manual brushes. Differences between manual and electric brushes are largely a function of novelty except for patients with disability. For such patients, adaptations—such as extra large handles or electric movements—can be helpful. Studies of the Sonicare electric brush (Philips Oral Health Care) have suggested that it improves the cleaning of interdental areas over the use of a manual brush, perhaps because the use of a timer increases overall brushing. Studies of various toothbrushing methods have also largely failed to show any differences between various methods. Vibratory methods, such as the Stillman and Bass techniques, are as effective as the circular Fones method, the vertical Leonard method, or simple horizontal scrubbing. The "rolling" or "rolling stroke" method has been suggested to be less effective than the others.

Brushing is more effective when toothpaste is used. Toothpaste is an important carrier of fluoride or other plaque control agents. The abrasive in toothpaste is also important for removing plaque.

Patients are often taught that they must brush after meals or before bed, but these times are often inappropriate for their schedules. Although brushing at one time or another may be marginally more or less effective, we try to help patients find an easy time and make sure to tell them they can be just as effective as someone cleaning on another schedule.

Disclosing solutions help patients visualize plaque. We use them primarily in the office; the key is to use them at almost every visit no matter what the primary purpose. At home, bleeding after toothbrushing or toothpicking is an effective visual lesson. Research (Toevs and Lukken, 1990) points to bleeding as an indicator of disease.

To facilitate learning, we provide as many cues as possible when the patient first tries a task. In addition, we provide frequent and specific feedback, paying special attention to positive aspects of the performance. In order to succeed, some patients may need several demonstrations of proper performance. It is important to encourage them with positive comments. Negative verbal feedback tends to discourage their determination to master new skills.

A monitoring chart can provide personalized, concrete feedback. Major problem areas—plaque, periodontal pockets, and bleeding—are marked in red on the chart. Patients place it on the bathroom mirror at home or wherever they normally clean their teeth. The chart reminds them to clean and shows them where to concentrate their efforts.

Interdental Cleaning

Interproximal surfaces of premolars and molars accumulate the most unremoved plaque in patients who do not already practice some form of regular interdental cleaning. For those patients, clinical experience suggests that we have more success introducing toothpicks such as Stimudents® (triangular shaped toothpicks) than dental floss and

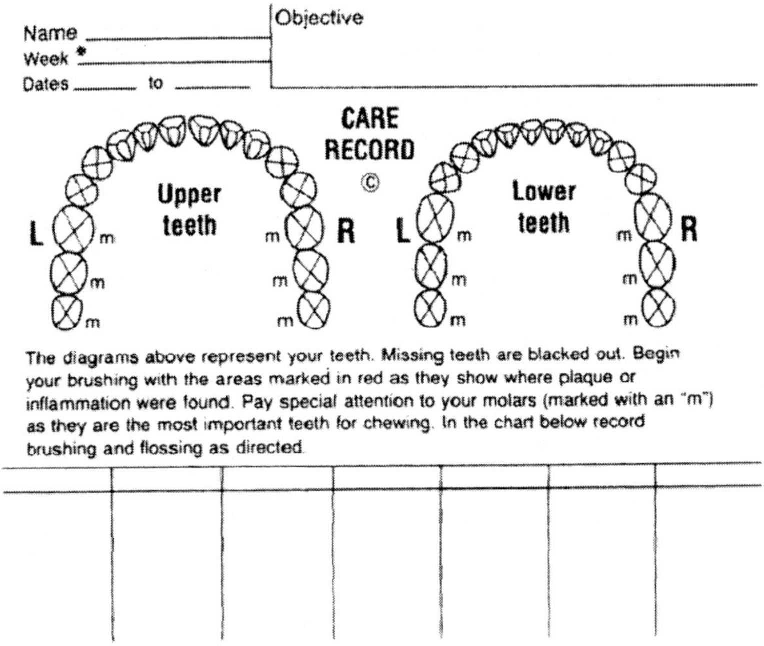

The diagrams above represent your teeth. Missing teeth are blacked out. Begin your brushing with the areas marked in red as they show where plaque or inflammation were found. Pay special attention to your molars (marked with an "m") as they are the most important teeth for chewing. In the chart below record brushing and flossing as directed.

tape. Toothpicks require less dexterity, and patients are more comfortable with the concept of using them. Interdental devices are good for demonstrating healthy and inflamed gums. We suggest that the patient select a site(s) to monitor; if it bleeds on tooth picking, she should record it. Patients can easily monitor their own progress with toothpicking. That is not to say that floss or other devices are unsuccessful. However, they maybe inappropriate for beginners in plaque control because they are technically too demanding. Some devices are clinically very effective (for example, interdental brushes) but require regular trips to the drugstore to replace tips that wear out quickly. Such a barrier may trip up even conscientious patients.

The choice of an interdental cleaning device depends on conditions in the mouth. Adults, especially those with periodontitis, have larger interdental spaces that are more readily accessible for cleaning than do children or teens. Also, toothpaste can be used with interdental brushes to enhance caries control. If there are problems with dexterity, a toothpick holder or even a floss holder may make it easier for patients to acquire the new skill. For some, the use of pipe cleaners or

Superfloss® may be helpful.

Interdental cleaning can be very important for a child with caries experience in the primary molars where the newly erupting permanent molar is in contact with the obviously infected primary tooth. In this situation the parent, rather than the child, should use a flat dental tape with toothpaste.

Feedback Is Important

Feedback helps patients perceive differences between the "old way" and newly learned skills. An important step is the transfer of skills from the dentist's office to home. A crucial step is helping the patient recognize the automatic nature of oral self-care. Although he may want to alter his behaviors, old habits often interfere. As a general principle, learning to make new responses to old stimuli produces "negative transfer." That is, the intrusion of old, automatic habits into new behaviors should be expected. To facilitate transfer of the new skill, patients must, for at least a period of time, make their oral self-care a conscious activity. Instructing them to look into well-lit mirrors (make-up mirrors are great) when they are cleaning without using toothpaste may be helpful, especially after patients have practiced new skills in the office using a mirror and the intense operatory lighting. Attention to whether or not an interproximal area bleeds is great feedback. Patients can easily learn to self-monitor their own gingival health.

Experienced clinicians are also aware that gingival bleeding can scare patients. Many will be reluctant to use interproximal cleaning devices because initially there will be bleeding from the gums. Often patients are unwilling to push the Stimudent or interproximal brush in between the teeth. Letting patients know that the bleeding will stop after a short time is important. Even so, for some patients a period of intensive professional toothcleaning and chemical plaque control may be needed first to eliminate severe gingivitis before the new habits will be welcomed. Another problem is floss cuts. Many patients are not careful with dental floss, and they snap it between contacts. This can result in nasty cuts. In this case careful instruction on how to hold and manipulate the floss and the choice of flat floss maybe preventive. This, however, is another reason to hold off on teaching these skills until other skills have been mastered and the mouth is healthier.

The most crucial aspect of any type of feedback is that it be given in a positive manner. This does not mean we ignore what needs improving; it does mean that we point out what the patient does right. Do you remember when you were a student and instructors evaluated your work? Which instructor was capable of getting the most out of you, the instructor who looked at your work and said, "Terrible. Why don't you..." or the instructor who said, "This looks very good. In order to make it perfect, why don't you...?" Do you see the difference?

Finally, we emphasize to patients that their new habits or cleaning skills do not necessarily need to take more time than they now expend. They can make substantial improvements by enhancing efficiency—that is, attending to undercleaned lingual surfaces and not overcleaning labial surfaces. However, the patient's ability to learn efficient habits from the dentist or preventive therapist does not ensure that these habits will be practiced at home.

Assignment for Chapter 5

Identify an adult patient, family member, or acquaintance who will agree to have you assess his oral hygiene skills and then provide training to eliminate deficits. You should plan for at least two short sessions with this person, about one week apart.

Below is a checklist to guide you through the assessment and training process. Plan at least 15 minutes for each of these two visits. Some learners find it useful to videotape themselves while doing these exercises.

Session 1

1. Explain the purpose of the session to the person
   - ❑ Gain permission to look at what the person does to see if there are any suggestions you may be able to make.
   - ❑ Discuss increasing efficiency (rather than adding time

burdens).

- ❑ Avoid negative comments and eliciting fear.

2. Assessment
   - ❑ Find a place where the person can brush his/her teeth with good light and a mirror.
   - ❑ Consider using a disclosing solution or tablets.
   - ❑ Ask the person to brush and do the best job possible.
   - ❑ Examine the person's teeth and make a chart of the plaque.
3. Teaching new skills
   - ❑ Focus on a particular problem area.
   - ❑ Avoid introducing new cleaning implements at this time.
   - ❑ Devise a plan while providing feedback.
   - ❑ Model behavior that you want, using aids.
   - ❑ Guide the person's hand/brush as needed.
   - ❑ Have the person practice multiple times.
   - ❑ Use cues such as counting (for example, brushing to the count of 5 before moving to a new tooth).

Session 2

1. Explain the purpose of the session to the person
   - ❑ This visit is for follow-up training. One short lesson is often not enough.
2. Assessment
   - ❑ Use disclosing solution or tablets to assess current plaque levels.
   - ❑ Observe problem area agreed upon at first session.
3. Teaching new skills
   - ❑ Focus on skills taught in the first session.
   - ❑ Don't introduce new concepts until you have evidence that initial skills are mastered.
   - ❑ Practice the skills introduced at the first session again as needed.
   - ❑ Provide positive comments, and avoid criticism.
   - ❑ Schedule additional sessions as needed.

Please note that toothbrushing is only one example of skills that may be taught during this exercise. Other possible skills include flossing, using mouthwash, or other oral health skills. It is important, however, not to introduce too many new skills at one time. Focus on one skill and do not move on to additional skills until the initial skills are mastered.

Part II:

Behavioral Technology

Exercises in Behavioral Techniques

Exercises in Behavioral Techniques

Chapters 6 through 11 introduce several steps for helping your patients make positive changes in their oral self-care or stop unwanted habits. As you read these chapters, we encourage you to do the assignments specified below that correspond to each chapter. This way, you are learning about the techniques and practicing them as you learn. We encourage you to try these behavioral techniques with yourself first, so that you are more comfortable with the steps when you present them to others.

Chapter 6 – Planning to Collect Baseline Data

Assignment 1a: Think of a habit that *you* have and would like to change. For example, do you bite your fingernails, snack between meals, or smoke cigarettes? Do you want to exercise more frequently, keep your work area neater, or keep better track of your finances? Being honest with yourself, what stage of change are you in regarding this behavior? What barriers do you see to changing this habit? What are the benefits to changing?

Once you have chosen a habit that you would like to stop or begin:

- ❑ Think about what data you would like to collect about this habit. For example, if you smoke, you might like to count how many cigarettes you smoke per day. If you want to keep better track of your finances, you can make notes about how many financial transactions (for example, stops at the ATM or credit card purchases) you make in a week.
- ❑ Come up with a "scorecard" where you can keep track of the baseline data. What will this card look like? Where will you keep it? How often will you record? How long will you record?

Remember, the focus right now is not on changing the behavior, just recording how often the behavior happens.

Assignment 2a: Identify a person (for example, a friend, family member, or patient) who would like to change an oral-health-related habit. For example, your friend may want to start flossing more often, or you may have a patient who would benefit from more frequent toothbrushing.

- ❑ Be sure to use the skills reviewed in the Motivational Interviewing chapter to assess the person's readiness to change. Does he or she need to move farther along in the stages of change before you plan an intervention? If so, what can you say or do to help this person move closer to being ready to change?
- ❑ Once you have identified a person who is ready to pursue a behavior change, follow the steps above to think about what baseline data to collect and how to collect it.

Chapter 7: Specific Goals and Objectives

Assignment 1b: Now that you have collected baseline data about your own habit, look back on your "scorecard." What stands out to you? Are you surprised by anything you recorded? Looking at where you are now with this habit, think about where you would *like* to be.

- ❑ What is your *long-term* goal? For example, do you want to stop smoking or balance your checkbook every week?
- ❑ Think of some *intermediate* goals. For example, you can gradually cut down the number of cigarettes you smoke every day or write out a weekly budget. Think of these intermediate goals as steps toward the long-term goal, becoming more challenging with each step.
- ❑ Be sure that both the long-term and intermediate goals are very concrete, clear, and easy to keep track of. Avoid vague goals such as "exercise more every day." Instead aim to "take the stairs to my office instead of the elevator."

- ❑ Do you see any barriers to these goals? For example, do you live with a roommate or spouse who also smokes? Would bad weather keep you from exercising outdoors more regularly?

Assignment 2b: Review the "scorecard" the person has kept, and ask him or her: "What stands out to you? Are you surprised by anything that you recorded? Looking at where you are now with this habit, think about where you would *like* to be?" Be sure to use open-ended questioning to assess how ready the person is to change a particular habit before planning specific goals.

Follow the steps above to negotiate long-term and intermediate goals with the other person. What would the other person ultimately like to change? What steps do you both see leading up to that goal? Be sure that all of the goals are realistic to both of you, and that you work together to determine these goals.

Chapter 8: Planning an Intervention

Assignment 1c: Review your long-term and intermediate goals, and come up with a specific "road map" for reaching these goals. Issues to address are:

- ❑ What is your motivation for changing this behavior? It may be helpful to write down this goal or have a picture or other object to remind you of the long-term goal.
- ❑ What barriers do you see to each step of the behavior change? For example, if you are trying to stop snacking between meals, and you typically go for a mid-morning "coffee break" with co-workers, how will you navigate this challenge?
- ❑ How will you record your progress?
- ❑ How much time will you plan for each intermediate step?
- ❑ What reinforcers will you use? When will you receive the reinforcers? What will you do if you don't reach a goal?
- ❑ Will you tell others about your plan? How involved will they be in your behavior change (for example, will they "check in" with you regularly to keep you on track)?

Assignment 2c: Now that you have established a set of goals, negotiate a "road map" with this person about the specifics of the intervention. Be sure to work with the patient to negotiate the specifics. Assess barriers to each step. In addition to the steps listed above, be sure to discuss these details:

- ❑ How often will this person check in with you about progress?
- ❑ Will this person be responsible for giving him/herself reinforcers, or will you be involved? This may be especially important if you are working with a child. For example, if the child is trying to brush more often, both you and the parents should be reinforcing this behavior with social and/or material reinforcers.

Chapter 9: Monitoring and Modifying the Plan

Assignment 1d: Once you have begun to take steps to make a change, it is important to take an honest look at how you are doing with your behavior change. Sometimes problems come up almost immediately. Are you moving through the steps at the rate you had previously planned, or have things stalled along the way? Important questions to ask yourself are:

- ❑ Has my level of motivation changed from when I started? If so, why? What stage of change am I in, and what would need to change for me to be more ready for this plan?
- ❑ What has gotten in my way of making this change? Are family, work, or social factors impeding my progress?
- ❑ Are the goals and reinforcers that I set up working? Are they too easy or too difficult to reach? Am I really allowing myself these rewards only if I reach my goals, or am I rewarding myself even if I don't reach my goals?
- ❑ Are there other changes that I should make to the plan?

Assignment 2d: When you are monitoring another person's behavior change plan, be sure to avoid judgmental or critical statements. Remember that you and the other person worked on this plan together, and you both hold responsibility for its success. In addition to the questions listed above, be sure to ask how you might be able to help the person further in achieving the goals. For example, does the person want you to make "reminder" phone calls? Negotiate modifications to the plan as needed.

Chapter 10: Maintaining Change

Assignment 1e: By this time, the change you have made should feel more "routine" than when you first started. This is a good time to go back and review your baseline data "scorecard" and your written records of your progress to remind yourself how far you have come. It is also time to start "phasing out" the reinforcement schedule while maintaining a self-monitoring system.

- ❑ What changes in reinforcements would likely be effective for you? Should you make the reinforcements less frequent or harder to achieve?
- ❑ Are there things about your behavior change that are reinforcing themselves (for example, your fingernails may look so much better after you stop biting them that you are constantly reinforced not to bite them)?
- ❑ What can help you avoid relapse? For example, you may want to set up weekly or monthly check-ins with another person or put a "before" picture up on your refrigerator.
- ❑ Are there other changes you would like to make that could build on the change you've already made? For example, if you have lost some weight, you may want to start working out in a gym to tone your muscles.

Assignment 2e: This is the time to review the progress the person has made and discuss "phasing out" reinforcements. As in all the previous steps, it is very important to negotiate this phase with the other person so that the decisions are acceptable to both of you. Ask the person the same questions above, as well as how they feel about the change that they have made. Be sure to use social reinforcement of your own to encourage the person to maintain this change.

"Half of our mistakes in life arise from feeling where we ought to think, and thinking where we ought to feel.

J. Collins"

Chapter 6

Planning to Collect Baseline Data

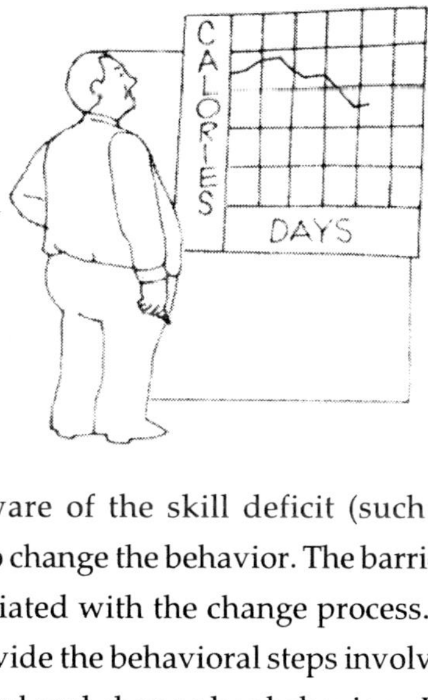

Earlier in this book, we reviewed the concept of Motivational Interviewing, in which we described how to assess a patient's readiness to change behavior. The next several chapters provide further details about problem solving and planning to help your patient change. As previously discussed, when the patient is in the *contemplative* stage, she is aware of the skill deficit (such as inadequate brushing) and desires to change the behavior. The barriers to change are the difficulties associated with the change process. In the following chapters, we will provide the behavioral steps involved in helping the patient move forward and change her behaviors. We will begin with an explanation of collecting baseline information.

Baseline Counting

The very first step toward beginning or changing a behavior with a patient who is voicing self-motivational statements is to assess how often the current behaviors are occurring. The best way to do this is to obtain *baseline counts*. Baseline counts are tallies of behavior or measures of current status, such as periodontal probings charted *before a* change is initiated. The most important reason for taking a baseline is that later on it lets you determine whether or not the change procedure you used was effective: you can compare conditions before and after the change procedure.

It might seem that any change in behavior would be readily apparent—that there is really no need for an objective verification that comes from taking before-and-after counts. However, often this is not the case. For example, consider the following case:

- At the initial evaluation, the patient presented with almost 75% of surfaces with plaque. The patient was given oral hygiene instruction targeting the anterior teeth and was reevaluated at a subsequent restorative appointment.
- At a follow-up appointment, a decrease in plaque of almost 25% had occurred, and a pattern had been established. Both the dentist and patient could easily have discounted the changes because the patient's performance is still far from ideal. Without baseline data to compare to current performance, the patient might have become prematurely discouraged and discontinued all efforts to improve or change.

This example demonstrates the value of gathering baseline data, particularly when there is a significant change to be made or when incremental changes are not readily observed by the patient.

Another helpful aspect of baseline data is that they often affect our thinking about the importance of changing a behavior. Sometimes, for example, it may seem as if a patient exhibits disruptive or annoying behavior all the time, or that a child never brushes his teeth. But it is often easy to overreact to certain behaviors and to overestimate their frequency. Taking a baseline helps you objectively determine the seriousness of the problem. In turn, this helps you decide whether or not you want to invest

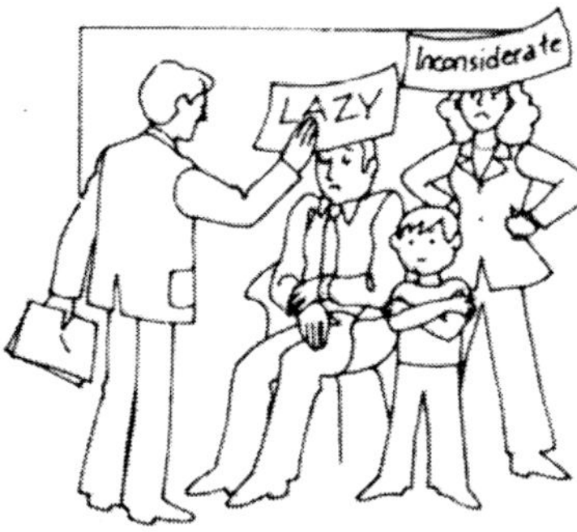

the time and effort involved in initiating a change.

Sometimes collecting a baseline results in a decision not to change a particular behavior at the time. Without counting specific behaviors, it is easy to over- or underestimate how often a behavior occurs. For example, you may find that a child patient is not as disruptive as he seemed to be— he misbehaves only during particular procedures (i.e., during injections).

Baseline counts will help you to set realistic goals. For example, for the motivated adolescent who wears headgear only two hours per day, aiming for her to wear the headgear three hours per day may be a useful intermediate objective. When she achieves a specified intermediate objective, she feels successful and is likely to attempt further progress. Unless you know how frequently a behavior occurs to start with, it is difficult to set realistic and meaningful objectives that will let you know when you have achieved your objectives.

Finally, baseline counting enhances awareness of a problem and movitation to solve it. In fact, baseline counting may itself lead to change. For example, counting the number of cigarettes smoked may lead a smoker cut down on smoking cigarettes during the baseline period.

Preparing to Count

Before you begin counting a behavior, you must describe the particular behavior in terms of when and where it does or does not occur. This is known as *pinpointing*, and it is the first part of taking baseline data. For example, if you are concerned about a patient's poor oral hygiene and have determined that the problem is in part a lack of performance, you would want to pinpoint when and where she brushes, as well as the depth of her periodontal pockets.

Pinpointing is important for the very practical reason that behavior change procedures are most effective with events that can be identified and directly measured. Consequently, it is best to translate your feelings or impressions about the behavior into pinpointed descriptions of it.

If you stray from behavioral observations, it is much too easy to attribute false motivations to others. Patients who do not brush regularly may be seen as lazy, or patients who arrive late for appointments may seem inconsiderate. These labels only get in the way of working with a patient. Remember, you are not trying to change someone's personality. You want to change only the behavior that is hampering good dental care. This can be facilitated by keeping in mind several simple questions:

1. What does the individual do or fail to do that brings about the problem situation?
2. In what situations, or when and where, does the desired behavior occur or fail to occur?
3. Is your description of the problem free of words which interpret, explain, or judge?
4. Can you count or measure the behavior you described?

In every case, your objective is to identify specific behaviors you would like to see occur more or less frequently in a particular situation. For example, you may ask patients to increase the length of time spent brushing each day or the number of hours per day of wearing headgear, or to decrease the number of between-meal snacks or the number of cigarettes smoked per day.

Engage the patient in a brief but important discussion of where and when the behavior in question occurs and does not occur. Please see the discussion in the Motivational Interviewing chapter for examples of ways you can introduce the idea of behavior change but avoid judgmental language. This sets the stage for making arrangements with the patient to collect baseline information.

Taking a Baseline

When is it necessary to collect baseline rates before trying to initiate a change? You must consider both the problem and the individual. Baserates are useful when *frequency* and *quantity* are important. For example, it may be useful to count the number of minutes a patient brushes or wears headgear per day.

With problems focusing on the *effectiveness* of a behavior, such as improving the percentage of surfaces brushed, a baserate collection period is less important. The age and character of the individual are also factors. Baserate collection is frequently very useful with children and young teenagers, or with adults who like or need structure.

Basic Considerations

In counting behavior, it is not always necessary for *you*, the dental professional, to count the behavior in question. There may be times when someone else is in a better position to do so. For example, a parent can be asked to monitor the toothbrushing behavior of a child between dental appointments.

To measure change, *rates* and *percentages* are calculated. When we say a behavior occurs once a week, eight times a minute, or six times an hour, we are making statements about the *rate* at which the behavior occurs. In contrast, when we measure the number of tooth surfaces a patient reaches while brushing, we are making statements about the *percentage* of the total number of possible surfaces or the number of surfaces that we have targeted.

Baseline Counting and Recording Techniques

If you decide it would be helpful to collect baserate data over a period of time, these data should be recorded in a simple manner, allowing you and the patient to see a pattern of behavior. There are several ways to keep track of behavior.

Event recording. Obviously, the most accurate counts are obtained when the behavior is recorded every time it occurs. *Event recording* is simply the process of recording the pinpointed behavior each time it occurs, using a chart such as the one below and then dividing the total number of occurrences by the time period to obtain the rate. As shown here, a patient is encouraged to write down the time and date of each time he brushes and flosses on each day during a two-week period.

Another simple technique involves the use of an object that can be

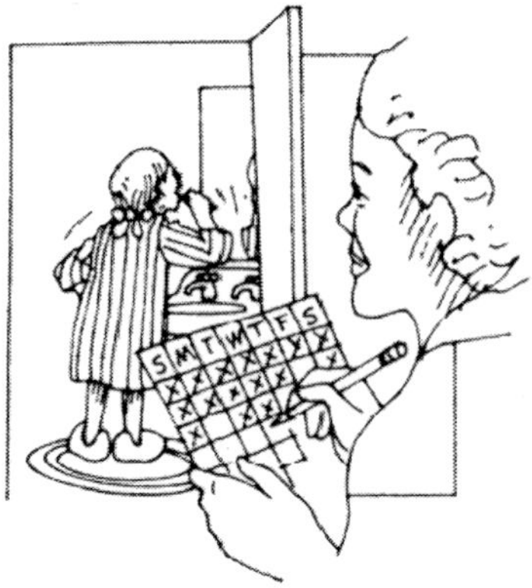

easily moved from one spot to another each time a behavioral event occurs. For example, a patient may find it helpful to move a paper clip from one jar to another each time he flosses, counting up the total number of paper clips moved at the end of the measurement period. For behaviors that occur frequently, however, such as nail-biting, this can be cumbersome, and patients may tire of counting before the end of the measurement period. Nearly any form of counting will call attention to the fact that a behavior is being counted. However, in behavior change, the idea is usually to make the person more aware of his behavior, and counting the behavior does this very well.

Time sampling. With some behavior, such as nailbiting or

Home Care Project

Name MS. ADAMS

Objective BASERATE - 2 WEEKS

Week	Sun	Mon	Tues	Wed	Thur	Fri	Sat
No. 1 Dates 9/7 to 9/13	B 9AM	B 8AM	B 8AM	B/F 7AM	B/F 7AM	B/F 6:30AM	B 11AM
No. 2 Dates 9/14 to 9/20	B 10AM	B/F 7AM	B 8AM	B/F 7AM	B 8AM	B/F 7AM	B 10AM

thumbsucking, practical considerations make it difficult to count every instance of behavior twenty-four hours a day. In such cases, it is customary to record events in a way that makes determining the rate as easy as possible. In using *time sampling,* you select a specific time period and count the frequency of behavior during that time each day. For example, a patient may decide to count instances of thumbsucking between 10 AM and 12:30 PM and between 4 PM and

5:30 PM each day. Thus, as in event recording, you count every instance of a behavior, but only for a limited period of time.

Counting the permanent products of behavior. The *permanent* products method can be used whenever a pinpointed behavior results in a concrete product that can be counted: for example, the number of cigarette butts left in an ashtray (or kept in a plastic baggie) or the number of assignments completed in class. When using this method, you can take a tally once a day or once a week and record it as a daily or weekly rate. When counting the behavior of another person, this method frees you from the necessity of being present whenever a behavior takes place.

Some Methodological Considerations

When you decide that collecting a baserate is necessary, it is usually best to have a person monitor his own behavior, because counting increases the person's awareness of the specific behavior. However, note that whenever a person is taking her own baserate data or is aware that her behavior is being recorded, the behavior will tend to either decrease or increase in frequency, depending on the desired results. In other words, *baseline recording tends to affect the rate of behavior when the individual is aware that recording is taking place.* For example, when a person begins recording the number of cigarettes he smokes each day, it is not surprising that the number drops off day by day. As previously noted, **just increasing awareness through counting can often be an effective method of helping a person to alter his or her behavior.** In some cases taking baserate data will act as a strong enough "intervention" to result in a change in behavior patterns.

Thus, in situations where the person is aware of baserate counting, *it is important that the baseline period be long enough to obtain an accurate count before the formal intervention plan is begun.* This is because many people revert to the established pattern once the novelty of recording wears off. In some situations the baseline counting can be done without the individual's awareness, such as when a parent records a child's toothbrushing frequency. Then what is called a "true" preintervention baserate can be obtained.

How long should you take baserates counts? They are generally taken for five to 14 days before you implement a change procedure. This observation period provides you with a good idea of a behavior's frequency and enables you to decide what you'd like to see happen to that behavior and to set reachable intermediate goals. Finally, it also gives you an opportunity to address any problems that may arise in counting or reading. For example, you may discover that your counting method is too obtrusive or too inconvenient.

Even though you will find yourself eager to begin the change procedure, it is extremely important neither to skimp on baserate counts nor to estimate frequency. Patients are sometimes tempted to estimate counts in order to produce results they think you want to see. Consequently it is important to emphasize to the patient that there is no right, wrong, or judgment involved. You must make it clear that a major reason for the failure of many projects lies in an insufficient or inaccurate baserate. If you do not have a clear idea of what a behavior is like before you try to change it, how can you evaluate the effectiveness of your change procedures and correct any mistakes you might be making?

What if a Patient Doesn't Record?

As we have seen in earlier chapters, it is critically important for patients to "be on the same page" as the dental professional during all phases of behavioral change, including measuring baserates. It is possible that after agreeing to measure baseline data, a patient will return for the next appointment with little or no data to show. At this time, it is very important not to be judgmental toward the patient nor to assume that "there's no point" in attempting further behavior change. If a patient does not complete the recording task, engage him in a problem-solving discussion about the task. Do not assume that simply because he did not complete the task he does not wish to change the behavior in question.

For example, a patient may explain that she placed the record sheet in an inconvenient place and forgot to use it. In this case, you may suggest keeping the record sheet in the bathroom (for recording toothbrushing or flossing) or wrapped around a cigarette pack (for recording numbers of cigarettes smoked). If the patient says he didn't have time to record during the day, have him set up a time at the beginning or end of the day to record. If necessary, review with the patient why he or she wants to change the behavior in question (please see the Motivational Interviewing chapter for how to elicit self-motivating statements). Simply lecturing the patient as to why you, as the dental professional, think she should change will produce resistance and set up both parties for failure.

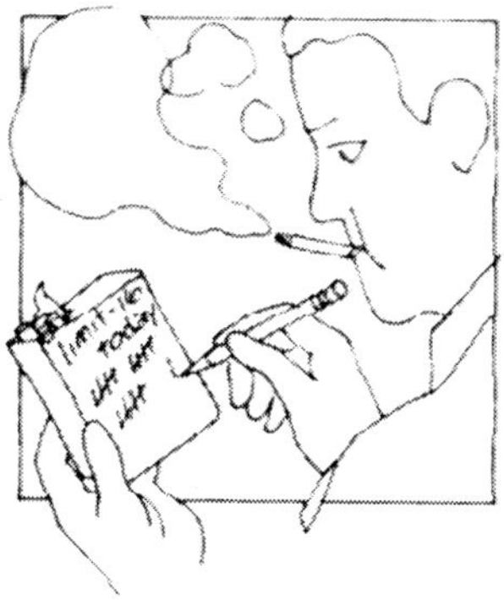

The Importance of Charting

Whether you are taking a baseline measure or attempting to implement change procedures during the intervention phase of the program, it is important to keep good records in chart form. Records, like a temperature gauge, show you small changes that ordinarily would not be noticed or appreciated. They also serve as an important source of motivation and reinforcement for everyone concerned. For example, a hygienist might wish to be able to check the progress of his plaque control program through a review of a child's record of the frequency and time spent brushing, or rinsing with fluorides. Even though no dramatic changes in the patient's dental health may occur immediately, he can see an objective improvement in his oral health care habits, and can be reinforced for these changes. The illustration on page 129 shows an example of how a patient's cigarette smoking decreases over time during the recording period. Without this written record, the patient may not realize the steady decrease in smoking and may become frustrated.

A good chart of improvements serves to detect even small improvements in behavior. In fact, self-control and self-modification procedures depend largely upon the use of *shaping* and charting skills.

Home Care Record

Name ______________________________

Objective ______________________________

Week # __________ Dates __________ to __________

We will discuss the concept of *shaping* in detail in the following chapters.

The chart shown page 124 can be used to provide feedback on performance, and then taken home to serve as a reminder of where to place special emphasis. The chart shown above is more general and can be modified as needed for different behaviors. Patients are asked to fill out these charts and bring them for review at their next appointment. They provide a concrete basis upon which to plan and design appropriate intervention strategies.

Keeping a Diary

Up to this point, we have talked about baserate data gathering only in terms of rate and frequency. Keeping a diary is another aspect of this process that is very useful when an individual is trying to modify his own behavior outside the dental office. Besides simply recording frequency, he can also record the number of times he *thought* of the behavior. For example, he may record the number of times he thought of smoking but resisted, or the number of times he remembered to clean under his bridge but did not do so.

The patient can also record, in a log or diary, how he felt at the time of the recorded behavior. Obtaining subjective feelings and impressions can help patients see how they really feel about what they are doing. The following examples were collected by our students who attempted to help friends and patients stop smoking.

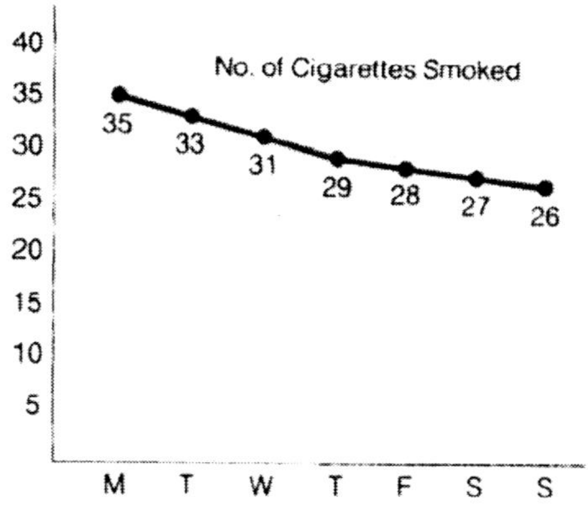

"I know this is supposed to just be the baseline period, but when I saw that I'd already smoked ten cigarettes and it wasn't even 1 a.m., I just put the pack back in my pocket."

"It's too hard to write down every time I do this."

"It really feels good to have a cigarette after breakfast."

Comments about the thoroughness of home-care activities may be revealing. For example:

"I finally had time to do a good job."

"I feel like I'm just going through the motions."

"At least my breath smells OK."

Such information may prove vital in helping you work with the patient to design a realistic intervention that has a greater chance of success.

A patient who is concerned about such problems as chronic headaches or other facial pain (such as temporomandibular joint (TMJ) pain, may record baseline data through a *pain log*. A pain log contains *quantitative* data, such as the intensity of the pain (on a 0-to-10 pain scale), duration, and time of day. It also contains *qualitative* data, such as how the patient describes the pain ("burning," "throbbing," "stabbing") and emotional reactions to the pain ("I just wanted to go go to bed for days," or "I was snapping at everyone around me.") Pain logs allow both you and the

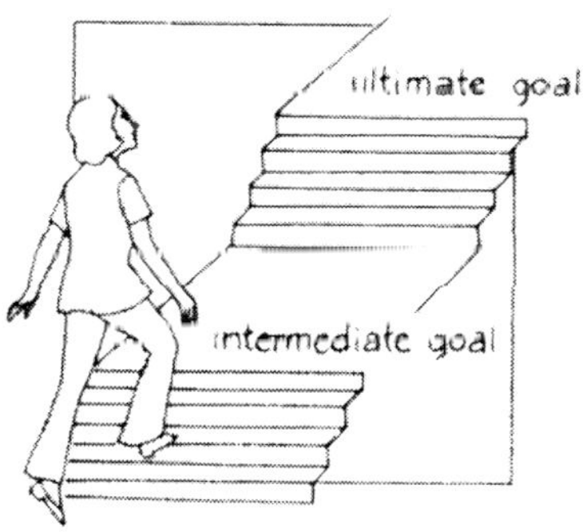

patient to assess changes in pain over time that may not be immediately obvious to patients as treatment progresses.

The Baserate Contract

A contract can be used to help solidify an agreement with a patient. Write up a contract, give a copy to your patient, and retain one for yourself. Often having a contract, which is simply a written statement of what you have both agreed to do, seems to make the behavior "more real" or "official." Children and some teenagers and adults respond positively to this type of structure. Patients will take the written commitment seriously and will usually attempt to live up to their end of the agreement.

This is not to say that a contract cannot be changed—it should always be open to modification. But any change should be a result of a discussion between the two of you. Contracts are most often used (1) to help clarify agreements to collect baserate information, and (2) to specify the conditions of the intervention plan once the goals of the program are agreed upon.

It is important to remember that a writing a contract is a technique that can be used to help both you and the individual you are working with to specify exactly what you want to accomplish and how it will be accomplished. It is not a tool to browbeat the patient into doing what you want him to do. Be certain to assess a patient's readiness to change before developing the behavior change plan, and be sure to involve the patient in deciding upon the behavior(s) to change.

Once you have collected a baseline measure or come to an agreement to collect baserate information, you have reached an end to what you can accomplish in that particular session. Between then and the next time you meet, the patient should practice the skills you have taught him, or collect baserate data, keeping a diary of his feelings. During the next appointment, you will either collect additional data (i.e., plaque scores) and provide feedback, or use the baserate information to formulate a specific intervention plan.

"Always do one thing less than you think you can do."

B. Baruch

Chapter 7

Specific Goals and Objectives

Once baseline data have been collected, you and your patient, now at the Preparation/Action stage, will have a clear picture of what is happening, such as when and where the behavior you wish to change is occurring or not occurring. You will then be in a position to discuss establishing goals and objectives for change. The specific methods you choose to control or prevent disease may vary. Sometimes, you may prescribe a course of antibiotics for a new patient with active periodontitis, or you may use a behavior change approach, such as when you ask the patient to begin brushing or flossing more frequently. In both cases you are concerned with devising a combination of strategies to solve a problem that will require active patient participation.

Choosing Long-Term Goals and Intermediate Objectives

We define goals as long-term targets. Although goals are useful in helping a person focus on what he wants, long term targets such as brushing and flossing twice daily or losing 25 pounds are remote and not easily achievable within a short period of time. By focusing only on the long-range goals, you invite failure.

As discussed in the previous chapter, it usually most helpful to focus on measurable *intermediate* objectives. Intermediate targets, or steps that "happen along the way," build up to the ultimate goal. For example, if you find from the baseline data that your patient is brushing more than 30 seconds twice a week, it would be unrealistic to expect the patient to start brushing for two minutes every day within a week. The goal requires too radical a change in the patient's behavior, and proposing this to the patient will lead to rejection and failure. Similarly, focusing only on the goal of losing 25 pounds ignores the much more crucial process of systematic weight reduction. Focusing on an intermediate objective of one to two pounds per week, or on even more specific objectives of consuming only a certain number of calories each day, are not only easier to achieve but also bring about more easily visible changes.

It is helpful to state goals and objectives in terms of behavior you want to increase, rather than focusing on stopping or decreasing a behavior. Thus, if a person is concerned about her nail biting, her primary objective might be "to use my nail clipper whenever I want to trim my nails," rather than "to stop nail biting." Note that in this example, the first statement is very specific, while the second is much broader.

Goals and objectives should be as *specific as possible*. Achieving "good dental health," for example, is a goal that is too general to be of use. When is good dental health achieved? How can it be measured? Such questions help in setting goals and objectives. A better goal might be no bleeding when brushing or using toothpicks. Here are some guidelines for setting goals and objectives.

Choose Appropriate Goals

When you help a patient initiate a program to break an old behavior pattern or establish a new one, you are using your knowledge of psychology. When people learn how to effectively change something about themselves, they strengthen and develop an ability that we generally call "will power." When people fail, their self-confidence goes down and they are less willing to try to change in the future.

Recall from earlier chapters our discussion about assessing patient readiness. It is important to obtain a sense of the patient's past experiences in changing his behaviors so that you can understand his ability and set realistic objectives. Obviously, the less realistic the patient is, the more effort you must expend helping design the plan and explaining the rationale behind a small-steps approach.

It is critical that the intermediate objectives be "reachable." Baseline data help you negotiate realistic objectives for that individual. What is realistic and reachable for one patient will be too difficult for another. If, for example, baseline data indicated that your patient wears his headgear three hours a day, three and a half or four hours a day may be a realistic initial intermediate objective. It is easy to be overly optimistic and enthusiastic in setting objectives.

However, it is also important not to "shoot too low." Setting goals too high will likely set a patient up for failure and discouragement. However, goals that are too easy to achieve are not likely to increase a patient's confidence and may lead to boredom over the slow progress of the behavior change. That said, it is generally better to err on the side of easier tasks initially, then increase the difficulty of tasks as patients achieve more success. Steady, step-by-step progress from objective to objective is slower than leaping to the ultimate goal in one giant step, but far more likely to achieve results.

Use Technology to Assist in Goal Setting

Dental professionals are extensively trained to instruct patients on the proper techniques for oral self-care, particularly toothbrushing. However, once patients leave the office, they may not "take to heart" your advice, or they may simply forget what they've learned. Research has suggested that although adult patients spend approximately 30-60 seconds brushing their teeth, or half as long as is commonly recommended by clinicians, they also tend to overestimate the length of time they spend brushing. Technological advances in toothbrushes themselves offer feedback to patients about the amount of time they brush. For example, some electric toothbrushes provide signals to indicate not only the "2-minute mark," but also 30-second time intervals to tell patients when to move to the next quadrant. A toothbrush whose handle changes color with the amount of time it is held significantly increases the amount of time children brush, compared to standard brushes.

When negotiating goals, it is important to be very specific. For example, simply encouraging a patient to "brush longer" is not sufficient, as the patient will not know exactly how much "longer" he or she should brush. Provide possible goals for behavior change, such as to brush "until the handle turns red" or "until the brush beeps twice," to ensure that you and your patient both understand the goals.

Get a "Jump Start" on Goals: The Chlorhexidine Example

Counseling patients to set realistic goals can be challenging. Because success depends upon individualizing a program for each patient, your knowledge of the patient's current behavior and your general familiarity with him or her are extremely useful. We have found in our clinical practice, especially with periodontal patients, that a "jump start" approach is often helpful. That is, with many changes the results are hard to see, and patients can become discouraged with slow rates of progress. Therefore, at the initial stages of instruction, we may prescribe twice-daily rinsing with chlorhexidine or a two-week course of antibiotics to help reduce plaque levels and clear up gingivitis. These are not substitutes for periodontal therapy or home care. Nevertheless, the results are often very noticeable and encourage patients to proceed.

Note that it is important to let patients know what you are doing. Tell them you recognize how hard it is to get started. When they return, praise them for following through with this approach even if their toothbrushing has not progressed much. It will help you maintain rapport and avoid guilt-oriented messages.

Here are some important tips for using chlorhexidine:

- Order and dispense an initial supply to avoid the problem of patients not getting the prescription filled.
- Write down specific instructions for use. For example, specify time. (Most patients will not remember to keep the solution in the mouth long enough to do much good unless they time

themselves.)

- Acknowledge some of the side effects, such as changes in the taste of food and staining, and discuss solutions.
- Have new patients try the taste of the chlorhexidine in the office. (If they are going to reject the rinse on the basis of taste alone, you should know it now instead of finding out afterwards.)

Similarly, recognize that there are limitations and even risks to the antibiotic approach. Some patients may not feel comfortable taking medications and will not follow through and get the prescription filled. Some will experience side effects and quit mid-regimen. Others will feel they have improved and will stop without finishing the drug regimen. Some will miss a dose because of oversleeping or a busy schedule and just not start again. Rarely do patients call us when they are unsure what they should do. Therefore, we always write down exactly what we want them to do and even make follow-up phone calls to see if things are going well. Experience has shown that such caring is perceived positively by the patient and is a practice builder.

Another way to accomplish these ends is to schedule a time for patients to call in and report how they are doing. Still another approach is to give them a post card to fill out and mail back after using the drug for a couple of days. However, antibiotics should never be prescribed without awareness of individual patient risk. In particular, the clinician must recognize the possibility of the patient's developing resistant bacterial strains and the fact that some patients are allergic to certain antibiotics. Sexually active females using birth control pills may experience increased risk of pregnancy when taking antibiotics. Consultation with the patient's physician and careful monitoring may be warranted.

Shape and Negotiate Realistic Goals

When we insist that it is best to work gradually toward only realistic, reachable intermediate objectives rather than focus on the long-range ultimate goal, we are discussing the concept of *shaping.* Shaping is the recognition and reinforcement of successful approximations in achieving a goal.

Shaping is simple and effective when (1) you begin at the level where the patient can succeed; (2) you negotiate intermediate objectives or steps, and positively recognize and reinforce the patient for his success in each step in the process; and (3) you move step-by-step in approximating your ultimate goal.

For example, if a patient has never flossed and does not regularly wear headgear or a lower partial denture, it would be unrealistic to expect her to make substantial changes—especially 100 percent compliance—during the first weeks of attempting to modify the behavior. Starting at her initial level of performance, you need to slowly shape her behavior and abilities.

One of the most common reasons a clinician flounders when attempting to change a patient's behavior is failure to use shaping. It is pleasant to think of receiving the positive consequences for immediate accomplishment of the ultimate goal. However, if the therapist recognizes the accomplishment of only the end goal or behavior, she will greatly decrease the chance that the patient will reach the ultimate goal. We must reward step-by-step approximations short of the ultimate goal.

Many people seem to be able to tolerate being an unskilled beginner in a new sport or exercise activity. They realize that results take time. However, others stop after a brief initial attempt. They exert themselves beyond their level of endurance in an attempt to get in shape, only to suffer muscle pain and an appreciation of their frailty. They push themselves to the limit to get fast results. "If one pill is good for you, then two or three must be better." "If running is good, I'll run till I drop." But results take time, and it is easy to end up saying, "I tried as hard as I could and it didn't do any good."

Similar situations may occur in dentistry. A patient with poor hygiene may brush or floss for a brief period. However, in the face of bleeding gums and some pain, she may become discouraged and quit. Another patient may brush intensively, mistaking firmness for quality, and may cause recession without improving his oral health. These patients are not building long-term health care habits. Instead, their efforts are to "get their teeth in shape," which is a decidedly short-term focus. Further problems, or the reappearance of symptoms after the intensive efforts have stopped, then lead to their thinking that they just have "bad teeth" or that "it's too much trouble" or "it really doesn't do any good."

Very frequently individuals resist shaping because they believe they should perform at certain levels and do not deserve to take pride in, or be reinforced for, performance below that level. This is an unfortunate attitude because it removes the possibility of reinforcement and learning. However, by shaping, a person begins at his current performance level and slowly but surely moves toward the ultimate goal, reinforcing himself as he progresses.

For example, in working with a patient to clean under a bridge, do not expect her to be flossing daily within a few weeks. Instead, shape behavior by negotiating and arranging reinforcement for flossing twice a week. Shaping can also be used to reduce or eliminate a habit such as smoking or nail biting. The statement "To hell with it, I can't do it" is frequently invoked. Such frustration is usually the result of trying to reach a goal too quickly and failing to shape behavior adequately.

A second problem that arises about goal setting is the issue of failure and success. Even if a patient accepts the idea of small steps, he may fail to recognize his progress or to reinforce himself for the changes he has made. Patients tend to become focused on the end result and discount the small but necessary accomplishments in between. At these times, forcefully point out, and strongly reinforce, your patient's *progress*. Do not let him get discouraged when he has not yet reached his ultimate goal.

Three Rules of Shaping

Rule 1: When in doubt, begin at the lower level. If you are having difficulty mastering a particular step, then take a step backward. In some instances, the step that you decided upon might be too difficult, and you may have to break it up into several smaller steps. For example, we often teach patients to brush just the upper anterior teeth before proceeding to other areas of the mouth. Be certain, however, that the goal you have set does not seem "too easy" or "silly" to the patient. It is very important that the patient see the step as being a valuable part of the behavior change program.

Rule 2: See that some positive consequences follow the behavior. In other words, plenty of reinforcement should follow each successful step. We will discuss reinforcements further in a later chapter.

Rule 3: Increase the difficulty—gradually, slowly, and steadily. Almost any program that calls for increasing some desired behavior should have a shaping schedule built into it. The following are two examples that utilize shaping techniques.

> *Example 1:* "I have found I am now studying approximately four hours per week. For the second and third week of my behavior change project, my goal is to study six hours per week. I will get the reinforcement only after I have done that much. This should be easy to do because I have done it before in the past. Beginning this week, I will require myself to study six hours" (in order to get the weekly reinforcement).

> *Example 2:* "From my baseline, I see that I am brushing only about four days a week. I almost never manage it on weekends or when I stay up late. For the next two weeks, I will try to brush every weekday and at least once on the weekend. I am going to move the time I brush my teeth to the morning.

Notice how the individuals in these examples followed the rules for shaping: start low, and keep the steps small. This allows them to enjoy slow but inevitable progress.

It is often tempting to create a time schedule as a motivator, but arbitrary calendar dates can impede your progress. Time schedules should be seen only as tentative guidelines. The rule for advancement is: Do not move up a step until the previous criterion is met. The study schedule in Example 1 discussed above has a potential flaw: The student may be tempted to move to the next level because it is week #2. He should not do so until he has met the first goal successfully.

In summary, the third step involves negotiating specific goals and objectives for the desired change. These should be small, concrete steps that can readily be identified. Recognition for the accomplishment of each intermediate goal and the progress being made is a crucial part of helping to ensure a successful change. In the next chapter, we will discuss such recognition in more detail in the context of planning the actual intervention.

"Many people fail because they conclude that fundamentals do not apply in their case.

M. L. Cichon"

Chapter 8

Planning an Intervention

Introduction

This chapter lays out specific strategies and intervention techniques for establishing new behavior. It includes strategies for either increasing the frequency of existing behaviors or decreasing the frequency of problem behaviors. As you read, keep in mind what behavior(s) you are attempting to change and try to identify which of the strategies you can use to achieve your goal.

We suggest you do not try to read this chapter at one sitting. Stop at the end of each section, put the book down for a while and think about what you have read. Before starting the next section, think about how the discussion might apply to you or to a specific patient you know.

The chapter is divided into three major sections:

Part A: **Increasing appropriate behavior by changing antecedents and consequences**

Part B: **Decreasing inappropriate behavior by changing antecedents and consequences**

Part C: **Summary**

In helping patients change, it is good to bring as much leverage as possible to the problem. This usually means using more than one technique or procedure to try to change the behavior. You might employ two or even three different strategies at the same time. The ideas and methods presented in parts A and B may be used in almost any combination to fit specific problems and circumstances. At this point we reiterate the crucial role of your personal expectations and enthusiasm in influencing the outcome of your preventive efforts with patients. Even when we receive an almost wholly technical service, such as when a grocery clerk rings up our purchases, we tend to respond more positively to a personal approach. Consider, then, how critical this element is in something as personal as the delivery of dental health services!

We are frequently asked, "How can I have positive expectations or enthusiasm about strategies I have rarely experienced, or with a patient about whom I have doubts?" The role most easily adopted by health professionals and with the widest acceptance by patients is that of *coach.* Just as a coach will try many techniques in an attempt to improve an athlete's performance, so, too, must you help your patient try out different strategies to see which ones can actually influence what he or she does. And, just like a coach, you know some patients learn more quickly than others but that repeat lessons are usually necessary. Your goal is to help the patient accomplish the goals he or she has already set, ideally with your guidance and input.

Part A. Increasing Appropriate Behavior by Changing Antecedents and Consequences

Two principles underlie all procedures used in changing behavior. The first is that *all behavior is learned.* Sometimes learning experiences are structured, as when we go to school or take a continuing education class. At other times, learning is a result of trial and error, as when we teach ourselves to ride a bicycle. Learning can also take place unintentionally— we may not even be aware that learning has taken place. For example, as children we eventually learn to mimic many of our parents' behaviors.

The second principle is closely related: *An individual's behavior is a function of his environment.* In other words, the behavior a person exhibits in any situation depends a great deal on that situation. For example, we all act differently with patients than we act among relatives and friends.

Antecedents and Consequences: How They Affect Our Behavior

Our circumstances clearly influence what we do. These circumstances are:

A. Antecedent **conditions of the behavior**
B. The pinpointed **behavior** we wish to alter
C. **Consequences** of the behavior

On the basis of thousands of observations and experiments, behavioral scientists have found that the events that have the greatest effect on a behavior are those that occur just before the behavior is exhibited (*antecedents*) and those that occur just after (*consequences*). By modifying either the antecedents or consequences, we provide a person with learning experiences and supply new information about what will follow a particular behavior.

For example, when we distract a fearful child, obscure his view of the needle, or tell him to expect a little feeling "like this" while pinching him, we are altering *antecedents* or what happens before the child responds to the injection. When a child is told she is being a "good helper" in keeping her mouth open wide, we are altering the *consequences* of responding appropriately to the injection. Strictly speaking, antecedents and consequences do not cause behavior; however, over a period of time, the repetition of a particular consequence in the presence of a particular behavior results in a very strong connection between the behavior and the events surrounding it.

Some consequences *strengthen* behavior; that is, they increase the probability that the behavior will occur in the future. Other consequences *weaken* behavior; they decrease the probability that the behavior will be repeated. **Generally, the consequences immediately following a behavior are considered to be the most important factors influencing the strength of that behavior.** Thus, most change procedures emphasize altering consequences.

Most people intuitively recognize that the consequences of today's behavior affect the way we behave tomorrow. This recognition is embodied in the system of rewards and punishments used by families, schools, and business organizations. Even though we usually recognize how much the reinforcement system influences our behavior, we often forget that we are always providing consequences for other people's behavior, even when we are not handing out reprimands, gold stars, or pay raises. In other words, we are continually teaching people how to behave, often without being aware of what we are doing or of the effect we have on others. If we often run behind on appointment schedules, patients soon learn that ten o'clock really means 10:25, or even 10:40. Every time we praise, ignore, reject, or criticize a patient, chances are we are teaching that patient something that will affect his or her future behavior.

It is important to remember that consequences affect the likelihood that a behavior will happen because the individual finds the consequences that follow the behavior either desirable or undesirable.

We cannot always predict what effect a particular consequence will have. The consequences that would increase our own behavior may weaken someone else's. Further, the consequences do not always have the effect we desire, and the effect may in fact be opposite from what we intended. For example, it is not uncommon to find that a loud bawling out or a spanking actually increases the behavior for which a child was reprimanded. In such instances, punishment seems, from the neglected child's viewpoint, to be a desirable consequence, because he can only attract parental attention by misbehaving.

It is important to remember that consequences affect the likelihood that a behavior will happen because the individual finds the consequences that follow the behavior either desirable or undesirable.

Antecedent Conditions of the Behavior

Identifying the observable antecedents and consequences of a behavior or habit can go a long way toward facilitating change. By identifying and changing these events, we can significantly affect the strength of that behavior in a relatively short period of time.

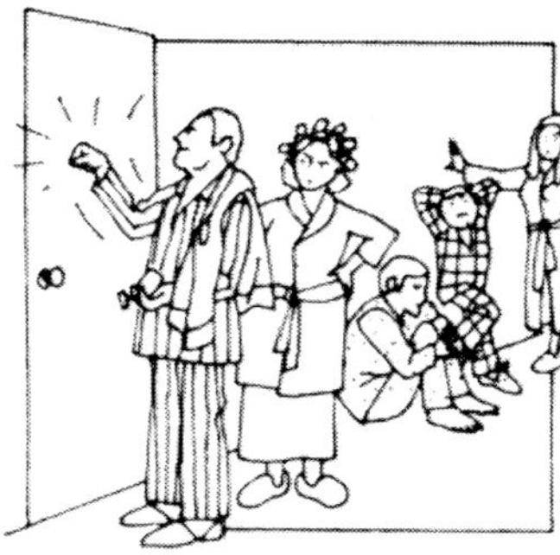

A good time to look for antecedents and consequences is when you or your patient are taking baseline counts of a behavior. Although your patient might try very hard to change, the situations in which he finds himself may make change all but impossible. Obstacles often arise that interfere with what your patient wants to do.

For example, a patient may find that no matter how much earlier he gets up in the morning, there is always one more thing to do to help the children get off to school. There is never enough time to brush carefully. Other people may also get in the way. In some households, there may be a lineup every morning in front of the bathroom. In such circumstances, the conscientious individual who desires to brush and floss may, in fact, be punished for his or her conscientiousness.

Identifying and eliminating, or minimizing, such obstacles may be all that is needed to provide a clear path to change. An effective intervention in such situations would involve helping the patient find a better time and/or place to brush and floss so that these activities would not interfere with his other activities or the activities of others. Such problem solving occurs when patients are at the contemplative stage and are preparing to act.

In some respects, observing antecedents and consequences is as much an art as it is a skill. The more experience you have with a particular patient or with a particular problem, the more adept you will become at discovering what types of events exert the most influence on the behavior in question.

There will be times, of course, when the events that control a behavior are not observable. A person's own thoughts may sometimes be the most significant antecedent or consequence of a particular behavior. For example, a patient with poor oral health may have intentions of brushing more often but may find herself thinking, "My husband *never* brushes and has never had one cavity! Why should I have to work so hard?" This thought may bring about feelings of frustration and may keep her from brushing as previously planned. However, the patient may not be able to identify these thoughts, making it difficult for you, as the dental professional, to identify the antecedents of the patient not brushing.

Even if you cannot easily identify the antecedents or consequences surrounding the behavior, you can still proceed with the behavior change program. The antecedents and consequences that you provide or that you help the patient build into his routine will be observable and countable, and you will be able to assess their effects on the behavior.

Using Antecedents to Change Behavior

Antecedent events may affect behavior not because they are desirable or undesirable in themselves but because, through experience, the patient has associated the antecedents with particular consequences. Antecedents can best be thought of as *cues* or *signals* that a particular type of consequence will follow a particular behavior. For example, to a motorist the sight of a police car is a cue that the consequence of speeding will be a ticket. To many people, the sight or smell of food — or the very thought that there is a goody in the refrigerator — may be a cue to snack.

As we learn to associate certain types of consequences with certain behaviors, the antecedent situations that are the cues to those consequences come to exert a powerful effect. When a motorist spots a police car (the cue), the response to slow down is often automatic. Just the sight of the police car causes the person to reduce speed. Similarly, many patients open their mouths wide when the dental practitioner approaches, without his saying anything.

Rearranging and controlling antecedents can be useful in the dental office. Even time may be used as a cue. For example, a child may be shown an egg timer and told that if she sits still until all the sand runs out, she can play with the suction device, hold her bear, or see her treasure that she will get at the appointment's end. Time structuring may also prove useful for anxious adult patients. For example, counting to ten and stopping for a rest during the drilling phase, or stating that the patient will be able to sit up in about five minutes after the tooth is prepared, can be very helpful for this type of patient. Such structuring of the dental appointment allows the anxious patient to pace himself.

When helping a patient establish a regular oral hygiene habit, you may find that there is no time pressure or other interference, but that the brush and toothpaste are kept in the medicine chest – "out of sight, out of mind." In such a situation, no antecedent cues to brush are apparent. It is not always necessary to make wholesale changes in the antecedent situation. At times, all that is necessary is to arrange for an antecedent cue to occur regularly in order to help remind the person to perform the desired behavior. Placing the brush and toothpaste or interdental brush in a highly visible place provides a cue for the behavior you are trying to increase. Taping a monitoring chart to the bathroom mirror can also serve as a strong reminder. Such cues help us by triggering our memory or by not allowing us to conveniently forget. We also believe cues need to be changed regularly; the same cues seen every day may soon be ignored.

Rearranging the Cues and Sequence of Events

This strategy is related to what is called the *Premack Principle,* named after the psychologist who studied the phenomenon. To help remember how this principle works, many people think of it as "Grandma's Law." Grandmothers are known to say, "First you eat your carrots, and then you can have your dessert." Any behavior that has a higher probability of being performed (eating dessert) can be used to reinforce any behavior of lower probability (eating vegetables) by making it depend on performance of the less frequent behavior.

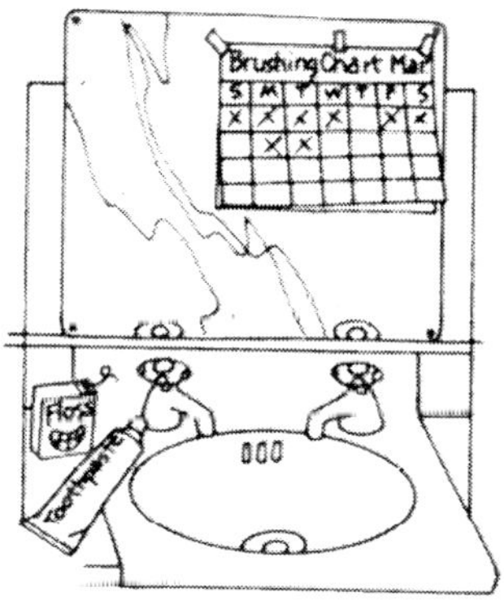

For example, though most people shower or wash their face every morning, they are less likely to brush or floss their teeth. If you want to increase the probability of a patient's attention to these home-care behaviors, you can do so by arranging events so that bathing or washing is dependent upon first brushing and flossing. That is, make an agreement that the patient will not bathe until after she has brushed and flossed. Here, washing or bathing is the more frequent behavior; oral hygiene the less frequent behavior. Similarly, if a patient always brushes, recommend that he floss before brushing. Note that the existing behavior to which the new, desired behavior is now tied does not have to be pleasurable or thought of as a "reward" by the patient. The primary criterion is that it simply be an existing, consistently performed habit.

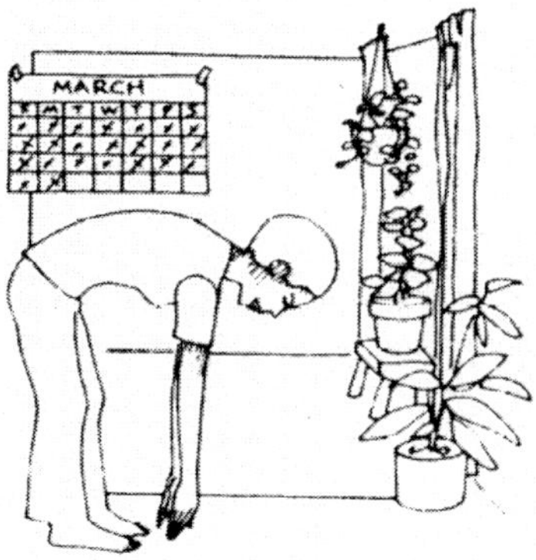

In using "Grandma's Law," we are altering the sequence of existing events. Anything we do on a frequent, consistent basis is reinforcing in some way. Such events often occur naturally, and it is not always necessary to create new reinforcers in order to strengthen a particular behavior. Some further illustrations:

> A young woman wanted to increase her exercise frequency from three to five times per week. A daily behavior for her was caring for her houseplants. She simply arranged events so that she would not care for her houseplants until she had done her exercises on selected days.
>
> A man who described himself as a "habitual jogger" made an agreement that he would clean thoroughly with his interdental brush before changing into his running gear.
>
> A government worker who started each day by reading his electronic mail was encouraged to use a Stimudent® around

his molars concurrently with the reading of the day's correspondence.

A student told herself that if she stayed in and studied "all day" Saturday, she would allow herself to go out Saturday evening.

This strategy can be especially effective when we try to establish a patient's permanent home-care habits. We are, in effect, linking the new habit we wish to establish with an existing behavior the patient regularly performs. In other words, we are weaving the new behavior into the individual's already existing pattern of everyday habits. However, merely tacking on a new behavior at the end of the day—for example, jogging after work or brushing just before bed—often invites failure. This is because when we are tired or under stress, new behaviors are the first to be sloughed off.

Using Consequences to Change Behavior

Changing the consequences of an event is the most common way to alter behavior. When we reprimand a child, give an employee a raise, thank someone for helping us, or give a student an "A" we are using a system of rewards and punishments to provide feedback that we hope will alter future performance in the desired direction. This change is the essence of the reward (or reinforcement and punishment) system. When we attempt to alter behavior by rewarding desired behavior, we are trying to provide positive feedback that is strong enough to encourage similar behavior in the future.

Providing Positive Reinforcer

What kind of reinforcers should be used? Since everyone is different, it is impossible to predict exactly what kind of positive feedback or reward will be strong enough to bring about change in a given individual. Let's first look at some basic principles in choosing reinforcers.

1. **Reinforcers have to have positive consequences for the individual seeking to change.** No matter how reinforcing

the consequence seems to you, it cannot be considered a reinforcer unless it increases the behavior it follows. People differ, and the reinforcers must have value to the person attempting to change. Thus, reinforcers must be tailored to suit the individual's needs and desires.

Sometimes an individual will chose a reinforcer that is rewarding for himself or a family member, such as a night out on the town, but which, because of the cost or inconvenience, actually becomes a disincentive to change. We have found that a reinforcer is most effective when it is something the individual truly desires but would not ordinarily treat himself to.

2. **Reinforcers must be relatively strong.** The more potent the reinforcer, the more likely it is to help change a behavior. One word of warning: It is our experience that patients can best choose what type of reward or positive feedback will help them change; however, adults are at first likely to choose weak reinforcers, such as an extra half hour of TV or some sort of "crackerjack prize." Encourage the patient to choose consequences she knows are actually strong enough to alter her current behavior.

   Consider this example: You are helping a child change a behavior by altering consequences. Perhaps you are concerned about getting him to brush, floss, or wear a night guard regularly. Unfortunately, although the long-range consequences for these kinds of behavior are positive, the immediate consequences are weak. And, as we mentioned before, it is very difficult to establish a new habit merely because it is good for you or because it has some other long-range effect. Thus, to increase your chances of success in establishing the child's new habits, it is wise to provide strong, positive consequences (or reinforcers) until the new behaviors become strong enough to maintain themselves without external reinforcements.

The easiest way to evaluate the strength or potency of the reinforcer is to ask, "Does the person seeking to change really think that she will change because of receiving this reinforcer?" Changing behavior requires work and effort, and most of us, when it comes down to it, are unwilling to work for a pittance.

3. **Reinforcers must be accessible.** You must be sure that any reinforcer you or your patient selects can actually be delivered. There is no point in deciding that $100 is an effective reinforcer if you do not have the money. You will be able to tell if a particular reinforcer is accessible simply by asking, "How will the reinforcer be delivered when the desired behavior has been performed?" Delivery of reinforcement, like behavior frequency, should be countable and monitorable. Kind thoughts are no substitute for observable reinforcers. In addition, they must actually be delivered.

Applying Positive Consequences in Dentistry

How do you go about selecting and choosing reinforcers in dental practice? The list of possible reinforcers is infinite. In identifying the reinforcers that might be appropriate for a particular person in a given situation, you will find it useful to consider three types of reinforcers: material, activity, and social.

Material reinforcers. A material reinforcer is any tangible item a person receives following the occurrence of the behavior that you want to strengthen. Such things are food, toys, clothes, money, or recreation equipment. Selecting a meaningful material reinforcer and devising a systematic reward system is frequently a difficult task. Except with young children, where we can use items from a treasure box, it is difficult for the health professional to provide or control any meaningful material reinforcers. The dental professional is not going to be able to come up with money or gifts as rewards. A second difficulty is that a program employing material reinforcers must be tightly and clearly structured in order to be effective.

We have found that the key to implementing a material reinforcement strategy is careful selection. It is necessary to explicitly discuss with the patient what might be used. Children easily accept working for rewards, but it is more difficult to utilize material reinforcers with adults. As we have mentioned, patients will often reject the idea. Alternatively, they might initially select "crackerjack prizes" (not significant enough to work for) or monumental rewards (hard to implement).

If possible, the reward should be something the individual desires, such as a night out with a special friend or a new dress, but not something that she ordinarily would simply go out and purchase. A system in which the patient actually sets aside the predetermined sum of money for each performance of the target behavior (or goal) is necessary to make the reward immediate and tangible. A patient can be encouraged to subtract the money from his checking balance without actually writing a check. Alternatively, he can physically place the money in a "cookie jar" following performance of the desired behavior. As phony as they seem, these strategies are helpful to some patients.

Activity reinforcers. An activity reinforcer is anything a person likes to do. The list of potential reinforcers is infinite, highly individualized, and includes such activities as watching TV, playing a game, participating in a decision-making process, talking with friends, or taking a walk—any activity that is enjoyed by the person being reinforced.

Two problems frequently arise with the use of activity reinforcers. First, patients will often suggest that they deny themselves some activity if they fail to perform the identified behavior. This is actually a form of punishment and is seldom effective. A more common problem is that people simply give themselves the activity reinforcer whether or not they performed the behavior or met the goal. This is especially true if the activity is something the individual likes and might ordinarily do. For example, a patient may decide to reward herself with a hike on the weekend and then find it very difficult not to just go ahead and go, whether or not she has reached the target behavior.

There are, however, several advantages to activity reinforcers. One is that they can be utilized frequently; another is that they are often inexpensive. They also often involve other people, who can add an element of social reinforcement, especially when they know of the project.

Social reinforcers. Social reinforcement can be thought of as any aspect of one person's behavior that follows someone else's behavior and strengthens it. The most common form is verbal praise, such as saying to your 8-year-old patient, "Judy, you are being a very good helper by sitting back in the chair like that. You are doing very well," or saying, "Ms. Domoto, three of the patients commented on how quickly you came to help them. I thought you would like to know." Hugging and other forms of physical contact are also forms of social reinforcement and may be appropriate to use with children. Commenting on a patient's efforts to become more interested and involved in his own health and reinforcing his sense of self-efficacy — an important element of the self regulation model of change — can be very helpful.

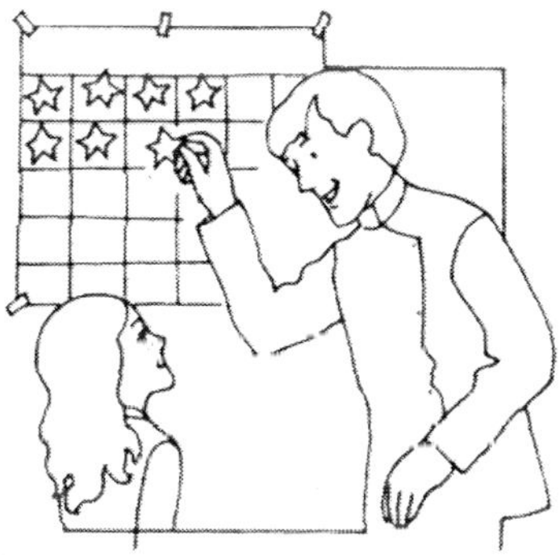

Social reinforcement is the most available, and in many ways the most effective, type of positive consequence or reinforcer. In addition to verbal praise, social reinforcement consists of anything you do or say to make a person feel appreciated, accepted, important, or just plain good. Approval, attention, and recognition in any form are usually reinforcing. Simply taking a few extra minutes to listen to people and indicating that you have heard and understood what they said can be reinforcing.

Because any form of attention may be reinforcing, be careful not to reinforce inappropriate or undesirable behavior by the use of criticism. After all, criticism is one form of attention. It is especially likely to reinforce undesirable behavior in those homes, schools, or offices where busy parents, teachers, or clinicians tend to notice an individual only when he or she is exhibiting an inappropriate or annoying behavior. Likewise, by ignoring appropriate or desirable behavior we simultaneously weaken it.

Feedback

One form of social reinforcement that is quite effective is feedback; that is, simply letting a person know how he is doing, and giving him information about how well he is performing in terms of a specific goal. Feedback is like a mouth mirror or disclosing tablet that shows a person the quality of his brushing. Bleeding when biting into an apple is also a form of feedback, suggesting that oral health could be improved.

Providing verbal praise to a patient during a long procedure is a way of increasing cooperation. You might say to your 8-year-old patient, "You're being very good at helping me today by sitting so quietly when I'm looking at your teeth." To an adult patient, you might comment on how much you appreciate his showing up on time for appointments. Notice that these two examples provide *specific* information to the patient about what the practitioner found helpful. General social reinforcement or feedback like, "Good," "You are doing just fine," "You are being a perfect patient" can and should be provided occasionally. However, such general comments do not let the patient know exactly what it is you find helpful. It is important to remember that the more specific you can be in providing feedback, the more likely it is that the feedback will have a positive effect on the patient.

Feedback can take many different forms. For children, and even for adults, making a mark on an attractive and well-displayed chart in the home or clinic may itself be reinforcing, even when no other consequences are provided. You may have noticed that towns, hospitals, and charitable organizations trying to raise money often post the current status of their drive, perhaps in the form of a thermometer or a tree sprouting branches, where everyone can see it. People are prompted to do things when they can see their behavior accurately represented in such ways. We have noticed in our own practice how many of our new patients have almost no idea about the nature of dental disease, or the effectiveness of their own efforts at prevention. Skills training can be very socially reinforcing if the dental professional's attitude is helpful and encouraging—like that of any good coach or teacher — and the patient receives multiple focused lessons spaced closely together with specific feedback on his hygiene skills.

Because feedback can be reinforcing, frequency charting often directly affects the behavior. For example, keeping a record of how many cigarettes you smoke per week may decrease the behavior in the desired direction. It is important to recall that when a person is aware baselines are being taken, he is likely to change his behavior, even if he is not yet really trying to do so.

What kind of reinforcer should be used? The distinctions between material, activity, and social reinforcers are not always clear-cut. For example, if a person rewards himself with a glass of wine for exercising, you might say that the wine is a material reinforcer, or that the opportunity to drink is an activity reinforcer. (Is it ethical to use wine as a reward? If the individual enjoys it, has no intention of giving it up, and is willing to let the habit be the reinforcer, should you impose your personal values about alcohol?)

Fortunately, it is not really important to categorize the reinforcers that you use to strengthen behavior. The reason for knowing about the different types is that it enables you to look at the patient's environment and ask three questions: What can be given, either by me or the patient, that might be reinforcing? What can either of us enable him to do that might be reinforcing? What can I or others say to him that might be reinforcing?

Using Reinforcement: Four Principles

Keep in mind four basic principles in designing a program to increase behavior:

First, when you have a choice of several different reinforcers, you should generally *begin by using the one that least disrupts the normal flow of activities and interactions and the one that requires the least amount of intervention*. Usually this involves using social reinforcement, which ordinarily consists of some form of verbal praise or feedback and recognition. It is often the most convenient type to deliver.

Second, *combine material or activity reinforcers with some form of social reinforcement*. That is, say or do something that demonstrates your recognition or approval. Using social with other types of reinforcers is important in any behavior change. It is really your goal to bring desirable behavior under the influence of social reinforcement and to eliminate the use of other types of reinforcers, especially material ones. However, using material and activity reinforcers together is often necessary in the beginning phases of a behavior change. The combination may continue to be the best method of reinforcement for young or persons with mental retardation.

Third, *be completely open with everyone about what you are doing*. After you have taken your initial baseline counts of the behavior, you and the person who you are working with should negotiate the reinforcement system, the plan of intervention, and the ultimate and intermediate objectives that you are trying to achieve.

Fourth, *be open to change*. The contract or agreement that results from this discussion should not be considered ironclad; it should be open to further change. Ideally reinforcement should follow every instance of the behavior you wish to change. This technique, known as continuous reinforcement, is especially important when you are beginning to establish a new behavior, or in instances where the individual whose behavior you are modifying is not fully aware of the consequences, perhaps because he or she is too young or is developmentally disabled.

In addition, the more immediate the reward, the more likely that it will have an effect. This is true no matter what kind of learning is taking place. If a golf pro watched you practice your swing but waited a week before providing feedback, its value in helping you improve your swing would be greatly decreased. Similarly, when a patient uses a reward to help establish a habit, the reward should be given immediately after each occurrence of the behavior. For example, if an adult sets up a system to pay himself $5.00 each day he uses floss and a Proxabrush, he should deduct that amount from his checkbook following performance of the behavior. Having the parent praise the child while he is brushing is another example.

Are Rewards Ethical?

At this point, you may be wondering if it is ethical to use rewards to get people to do something. Although people generally accept the idea that it makes logical sense to break tasks down into identifiable steps, accomplish them one step at a time, and keep track of progress, they sometimes balk at the idea of arranging positive consequences or rewarding themselves or others for their progress. They find themselves saying a version of, "After all, they oughta wanna do it because it's good for them," or, "We're not going to bribe anyone for doing what he should do in the first place."

Does arranging positive consequences for one's own or for another's performance constitute bribery? Let's look at Webster's definition of the word *bribe*. It is "...a gift or favor...promised with a view to...corrupt the conduct...of a person in a position of trust... ." Obviously, encouraging a patient to develop better oral self-care can hardly be construed as persuading him to do something corrupt.

We all perform some types of tasks for which we always expect some external reward. Wages, for example, are contingent on the work we accomplish, and we certainly don't consider ourselves "bribed" by our employer. In fact, a very common complaint among employees is that they feel that they deserve a higher wage for their efforts.

So when we employ a behavior management system to encourage children or adults to engage in an appropriate activity, it certainly is not a bribe but simply an arrangement to help them meet goals by recognizing and rewarding the efforts they make. For example, the extra bedtime story a parent reads each time a child masters a new skill encourages the child to work toward the goal and provides feedback on his or her performance. External reinforcers help provide incentive to a person who either has had little success in changing a behavior or has not yet developed internal rewards for the behavior in question.

External reinforcers, however, are designed to be used only in the initial stage of a behavior change program. The eventual goal is to direct the child or adult patient away from externally provided consequences and toward the intrinsic reinforcements brought by successful completion of a task. Once the person begins to experience success and the positive consequences for the behavior itself, the intrinsic, more naturally occurring reinforcers begin to be motivating by themselves.

For example, parents might arrange some special positive consequence for their child, such as watching television together or playing a game, if the child keeps his room picked up. As the child begins to realize the more subtle positive consequences of a neat room, such as being able to find what he wants and the decreased likelihood that things he treasures will be lost or broken, the original, externally provided consequence becomes less and less important.

A word of caution about setting up an intervention plan with a person in a family situation. It is important to spend some time inquiring about how the other family members feel about the individual's changing his or her behavior. This is especially critical if another family member is involved in the project, such as when a husband and wife both try to change oral care together, or when another family member is in charge of dispensing rewards or punishment.

For example, it may be that the other person likes things just as they are, such as when a husband doesn't really want his wife to stop smoking, perhaps because he has not been able to succeed himself; or one might use the charts to "needle" the individual who is trying to change (a frequent occurrence with parents and children). Make sure that both parties wholeheartedly agree to the conditions and that the terms are carefully written out and signed by each.

Finally, be sure to "check in" with patients frequently to assess the effectiveness of the reinforcers chosen at the start of the intervention. A reinforcer that helps motivate behavior change at the beginning of an intervention may lose its effectiveness over time. It is very appropriate to monitor and change reinforcers as needed to maintain behavior change.

Part B. Decreasing Inappropriate Behavior by Changing Antecedents and Consequences

We have discussed the effects of altering antecedent events and using positive consequences to increase the frequency of existing behavior. Now we will focus on the fundamental strategies designed to decrease the frequency of existing behavior.

Punishment

The first procedure we will discuss is the most familiar—punishment. Let's consider for a moment the concepts of punishment and reinforcement. Both are consequences that follow and change the frequency of behavior. The important difference is that reinforcement increases or maintains behavior, while punishment decreases or inhibits it.

It is important to realize that the same event that functions as a punishment to one person may act as a reinforcement to another. We have all been tickled at one time or another; some of us enjoy it, some do not. Sometimes a person likes to be tickled; other times the same person does not. It can be either punishing or reinforcing.

There is no absolute way of foretelling whether a specific behavior will function as a punishment or as a reinforcement. To determine this, you must compare the baseline record with the behavior after you have made your intervention to see if the behavior decreases or increases in frequency. If it has increased, we must assume that the consequences have been reinforcing.

Besides suppressing the behavior in question, punishment has a number of unpleasant side effects. First, we find that punishment often results in additional negative behaviors. Anger and uncooperativeness are typical responses. Second, when possible, the individual often will simply avoid the person applying the punishment. Many people avoid dentists and hygienists because in the past they have criticized them about the condition of their teeth or self-care. More likely than not, punishment is an inappropriate technique for health professionals.

Use of Punishment Techniques in Altering Oral Health Care Habits

Can or should punishment procedures be used outside the practice to change oral health habits? Intervention plans that rely solely on punishment seldom work, primarily for the following reasons.

(1) Undesired behavior is usually resistant to mild punishment, especially when it is applied after a delay. Punishment is most effective as an intervention when it is administered in large amounts immediately following the behavior. For example, not being allowed to see a movie would in all likelihood be too weak a punishment for not brushing. (2) Punishment usually results in avoidance of the punishing person and other negative emotional side effects that we mentioned earlier. (3) Punishment alone does not teach new or alternate forms of behavior. It often merely temporarily suppresses the behavior that precedes the punishment. (4) Punishment is generally effective in suppressing a behavior only as long as someone is around to administer the punishment. (5) Although interventions based only upon self-punishment may be effective, there is a strong chance they may not be enthusiastically followed. Most often, when choosing a punishment, people decide to take away some pleasurable event that is usually available—for example, an evening out or a favorite food. In the end, not all people will follow through on the agreement.

In some change projects, however, punishment by itself can be very effective. Some patients trying to decrease nail or cheek biting have reported that by snapping a rubber band on their wrist when they catch themselves performing the undesired behavior, they can decrease or eliminate the habit very quickly.

Clinical psychologists Nurenberger and Zimmerman (1970) reported an interesting intervention strategy that utilizes punishment. Patients agreed that if they did not achieve their objective they would mail a check, previously prepared, to the political or religious organization they hate the most. As with the use of other forms of punishment, it is best to use this device with reinforcement. As patients successfully reached their objectives, they rewarded themselves appropriately. Other psychologists have used similar procedures. For example, in an innovative experiment in 1971, clinical psychologist Hall and his associates reported that their patients agreed to tear up dollar bills or contribute twenty-five cents to charity for each cigarette smoked.

Now that we have explored punishment, a technique that is used only as a last resort, let us focus on some other strategies and techniques that can be used to decrease or eliminate inappropriate behavior.

Breaking the Chain of Events

We have talked about how antecedents can be used to increase behavior. Antecedents can also be used to decrease behavior. At times you may want to change the antecedents that lead to situations that you or your patients find difficult to handle. Many undesirable behaviors are the result of a fairly long chain of events.

For example, snacking may involve going to the supermarket, picking out cariogenic snack foods, taking them home, placing them in a convenient place, becoming bored or having nothing to do for a minute, moving toward the kitchen, opening the refrigerator or pantry, and finally eating the snack. By the time the person reaches the end of the chain of events, the impulse to perform the final, but undesirable, behavior is so strong it is difficult to restrain. This is particularly true for what are known as consummatory behaviors, such as eating, smoking, and drinking, where a behavior affects the consumption of the reinforcer and ends the chain. Such behaviors are very difficult to change.

Although change is difficult, a number of strategies that involve altering an antecedent event are effective in changing these behaviors. The first strategy involves a *two-stage process*. In stage one, the person deliberately avoids antecedent situations, such as parties where he might be strongly tempted to smoke, or dinner engagements where there will be a social obligation to eat a lot of high caloric food. During this stage, each time the person successfully avoids a tempting situation, he rewards himself generously. Social reinforcement in this situation can be particularly effective.

In stage two, a person rewards herself for being able to withstand the temptation even when exposed to it; for example, a repeated offer of hot apple pie at a dinner party. Three well-known organizations, Alcoholics Anonymous, Weight Watchers, and TOPS (Take Off Pounds Sensibly), use this strategy. Their primary reinforcement, based on social and interpersonal relations, is the approval, caring, and love of others for appropriate behaviors.

A second strategy is *early interruption of the chain of events*. Sometimes, by carefully thinking about the chain of events, it is possible to identify a weak link early in the chain. For example, one way of helping a patient control snacking behavior would be to encourage him to alter shopping habits. Another example may be the removal of vending machines in schools that provide only junk foods. If a "goody" is not immediately available, its absence enforces a pause—the person must either go to the store or bake from scratch, which helps break the normal chain of events.

Stimulus Control

Stimulus control is another technique useful for curtailing undesired consummatory behavior such as overeating and smoking. It involves arranging certain situations to provide cues for the behavior one wants

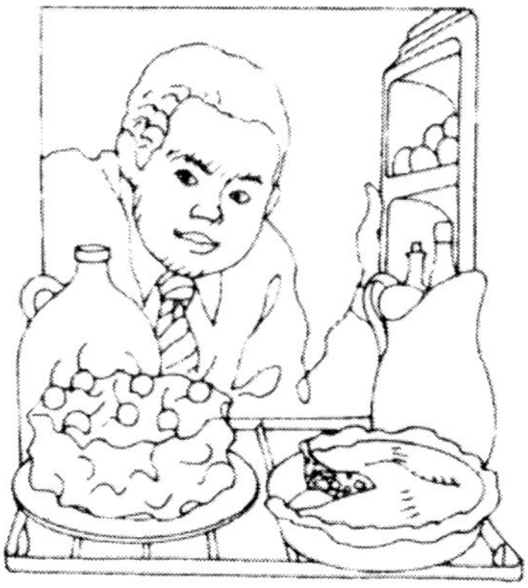

to control. Stimulus control and cuing can be used when elimination of the behavior is the goal. The logic is this: If a behavior can be firmly linked to an antecedent, that antecedent can be successively narrowed down in scope to the point where the behavior is unlikely to occur at all.

For example, psychologist Nolan reported in 1968 that a smoker agreed to smoke only in her "smoking chair" at home. This agreement restricted her smoking to a particular place; she no longer smoked at work or when she went out. Once she had established this habit, the chair was placed so that no other reinforcement besides smoking was provided — the chair faced away from the TV set, was not comfortable, and so forth. Once she had established smoking only in this location, she moved the chair out of the living room to the cellar! Under this plan, her smoking decreased dramatically.

Similar strategies have been used to control nail biting and are techniques that you and your staff might suggest to parents to minimize the ingestion of cariogenic snacks. That is, when children choose to snack, they will agree not to read, talk, watch TV, or engage in any other activity while eating.

Extinction

This strategy is quite different from punishment. Punishment involves presenting negative or unpleasant consequences after a behavior occurs. *Extinction* involves identifying the positive consequences or reinforcements that keep the behavior going and then stopping or withholding these reinforcements or consequences. For example, starting a meeting on time despite the absence of one or two individuals stops reinforcing them for showing up late. If the meeting never starts until they arrive, why should they show up on time? Similarly, when a child misbehaves in a dental chair, calling in the parent before completing a procedure may teach the child that misbehaving is a great way to get Mom to intervene. Moreover, if the child finds a parent's presence rewarding, episodes of misbehavior are likely to increase.

Typically, the initial results one obtains from applying punishment and extinction are different. When punishment is suddenly begun after every occurrence of a particular behavior, you are likely to see a dramatic but temporary reduction in the behavior. When reinforcement is discontinued, it is not unusual for the person to try even harder to elicit the same reinforcement as before. Thus, if the parent decides to start ignoring the cries of his 3-year-old, or when the practitioner does not stop what he is doing because of the whining of the child, it is quite reasonable to expect that problem behavior will increase temporarily. This phenomenon is called an *extinction curve.* When using extinction, you must be prepared for this phenomenon and have the patience to wait it out.

Using Incompatible Behavior

The procedure is similar to simple reinforcement. First you must identify an alternative behavior that cannot be performed at the same time as the undesired behavior. This new behavior is then increased through positive reinforcement to replace or substitute for the undesired behavior. For example, the parents of a 7-year-old who habitually sucked her thumb attempted to reinforce the alternative, incompatible behavior of hugging and holding her doll. This procedure is also useful in interrupting the chain of events that leads to an undesirable behavior. Instead of moving toward the kitchen, a person might "reach for their mate instead of a plate," make a phone call to a friend, or chew a piece of sugarless gum.

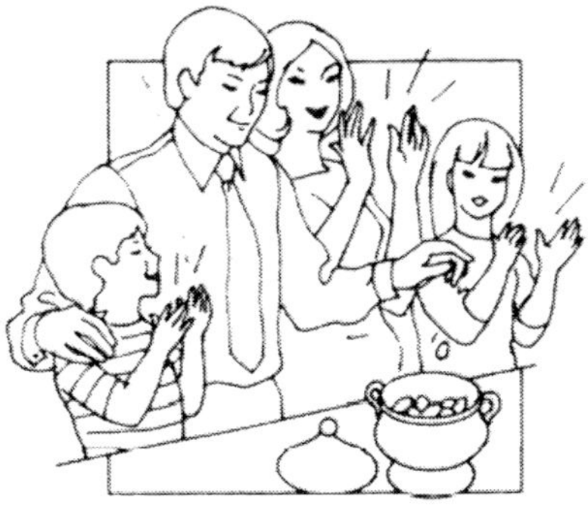

Experienced clinicians learn to ignore annoying child behavior that does not interrupt treatment, such as crying or whining, and to reinforce by praise and other positive consequences all incompatible, positive behavior, such as sitting quietly in the chair. Some smokers use the technique of substituting another behavior for smoking. Instead of lighting a cigarette, they take a piece of chewing gum.

However, mere substitution is rarely adequate. For the person addicted to tobacco, the value of gum compared to tobacco is quite weak. To increase the chance of success in changing, a person should also heavily and quickly reinforce the performance of chewing gum instead of smoking. He might, for example, make an agreement whereby his wife and family verbally provide support and encouragement, and deduct $5.00 from his checking account toward a new set of golf clubs as a reward each time he successfully substitutes gum chewing. Do not make the mistake of relying only on the performance of the incompatible response. An incompatible response must be reinforced or it will not be continued.

The reinforcement of incompatible behavior can be a very effective way to eliminate undesired behavior. This is because you are replacing the undesired behavior with a substitute. Here is another example of reinforcing incompatible behavior that will further illustrate this procedure.

Parent: "Dr. Richman, I'd like to talk to you about my teenage son, Sandy. Though he absolutely hates his dental work, and agrees in principle that it would be a good thing to stop eating sugary snacks, he has not stopped eating the snacks you said cause cavities."

Dental Professional: "Did you provide alternate snacks?"

Parent: "Both of us shopped for his favorite fruits, nuts, and vegetables. He knows that he shouldn't eat sugar snacks, but that's what he really prefers. When I see him eating that stuff and think of our dental bills, I explode. But that doesn't do any good either."

Dental Professional: "Well, simply substituting snacks may not be enough. Do you think you could reward him for eating other foods?"

Parent: "Reward him?"

Dental Professional: "Yes, instead of trying to convince him that he should prefer healthful snacks, provide praise, approval, and attention when he tries a new snack. You may also want to talk to him about setting up an agreement where you would provide special favors to provide incentive for him until he breaks the junk food habit, which is very hard to overcome. Want to hear more?"

Parent: "You bet."

This illustrates two techniques that go together: *substitution* and *reinforcement*. Another technique that could have been added involves altering the chain of events by having the parent refrain from buying any junk food to avoid having any readily available in the house. Fortunately, there has also been a recent movement in many schools to replace junk food and soda in school vending machines with more wholesome foods, fruit juices, and water. Encouraging more healthful snacks and beverages in schools makes reinforcing more healthy habits easier for parents and dental professionals.

The Problem of Cheating

Cheating by taking the reinforcer even though one has not performed the behavior is fairly common in self-modification. Almost everyone does it sometimes. If your patient is attempting to change his own behavior, you should sensitize him to watch very carefully for cheating. However, if he cheats more than occasionally, say more than 10 percent of the time, it indicates a shaping problem. One solution is for the person to require less of himself by attempting to reach the final goal more slowly. If your patient finds himself in this situation, the progression of intermediate objective should be redesigned so that he will be reinforced for performing at some level he finds possible.

Part C. Summary

You should now be ready to present your plan to the patient. The next two chapters discuss the last two stages of the change process — reviewing and making any modifications necessary, and termination and follow-up of the project. It is wise to bring as much leverage as possible to the problem. We strongly recommend that you choose or suggest *combinations of several techniques.* This is a crucial but often difficult step in the project.

Choosing and constructing a reward system that is actually strong enough to help an individual change his behavior is one of the most important and difficult tasks in any change project. It is important to remember how difficult it is for people to change their habits. Think of the last time *you* tried to modify your diet, lose 10 pounds, or implement an exercise program. Change comes slowly even with the best of intentions. The need for repeated "lessons" and reinforcement is the rule, not the exception.

In choosing a reinforcer, you are asking yourself or the patient this question: What, besides internal motivation, is going to be used to effect a change? What reward or consequence is strong enough to actually influence and change what you or your patients actually do? Glossing over these questions is the most frequent cause of failure in any program in which people are trying to change their habits.

The best time to begin attempting to identify reinforcers is when baselines are being taken. If you can determine the antecedents and consequences surrounding an event, and then alter them in some way, you will greatly increase your chances of success. When choosing a specific reward, it is critical to choose something the individual will *gain* if he succeeds at changing his behavior. The reward system should not be set up in such a way that the individual merely stands to lose something, or some activity, if he fails to meet his goals.

Sample Intervention Contract

I agree to do the following before my next appointment on (date):

1. Continue to post a 3x5 monitoring card on the bathroom mirror or wherever I brush/floss.
2. Keep checking off the boxes on the monitoring card right after each time I brush/floss for the period beginning (date) and ending (date).
3. Switch the time I usually brush/floss from just before I go to bed to just before I take my shower in the morning.
4. Move the floss canister out of the medicine chest and place it on the bathroom vanity.
5. Place a floss canister on the side table by my favorite chair to serve as a reminder.
6. Keep a daily log (a sentence or two) about how I feel the project is working.
7. Remember that my goal will be to brush every day and remember to floss every other day. For every date I floss I will write a check to myself (cash) for two dollars. This money is to go only towards a new metal tennis racket.
8. Bring the card to my next appointment.
9. Talk with Susan by phone on (date). I will see her for two 15-minute skills assessment appointments on (date) and (date).

Date __________ (Signed ______________________)

*(**Note**: The signature is optional, as it may be seen as coercive)*

If something can go wrong it will.

Murphy's Law

There is always a solution to every human problem—neat, plausible, and wrong.

H. L. Mencken

Chapter 9

Monitoring and Modifying the Plan

We have discussed the basic steps in developing a plan to help change your own or someone else's behavior.

Step 1: Assess your patient's readiness to change his behavior, including the motivation and any resistance to change. After establishing rapport and trust, ask questions, listen, and encourage self-motivational statements.

Step 2: Identify the specific behavior you wish to alter. Then determine whether it is the result of a skill deficiency or a management deficiency. The process of pinpointing is used to discover when and where the behavior in question is occurring or not occurring. Provide as much choice as possible.

Step 3: Take baseline measures or base rates to determine the frequency and rate of the behavior. This serves as a measure against which the success of the change project can be accurately assessed.

Step 4: Negotiate goals of the project, figuring out specific and realistic intermediate and terminal objectives.

Step 5: Again, with considerable input from the patient, plan and implement what will be done to help change behavior. Specify procedures, objectives, and rewards for successful performance.

Maintain an Active Watch

We will now focus on the sixth step—*monitoring* and *modifying* the intervention plan. Once the intervention plan begins, you must maintain an active watch to chart the program's progress and to work out any kinks or trouble areas. They will occur! It is not at all uncommon for some unforeseen problem to cause you to rethink and renegotiate an aspect of the project.

What to Do When Little or No Change Occurs

Problems occur almost immediately. The patient fails to pick up the prescription of chlorhexidine, forgets to post the base rate card, or says he didn't have enough time to practice a newly learned skill. At this point, the tone of your interaction with the patient is crucial. It is difficult to avoid failing into the role of "critical parent." Emphasize (as you ask, "How's it going?") that you do not want to be a critic or judge, but to work *with* him as a problem solver.

Recheck the stage of readiness:

As you'll remember from earlier chapters, it is very important to check with patients to assess what stage of readiness they are in at a particular time. If you do not see the changes that you would expect, this may represent resistance on a patient's part. She may not be in the active phase, ready to change. It is possible that after attempting to change, she became discouraged and returned to the Precontemplative or Contemplative stage. She may perceive too many disadvantages to changing in comparison to the perceived benefits. This is the time to take a step back and assess the patient's stage of readiness and engage in some problem solving with her.

Troubleshoot and reinforce:

If you are not observing any, or as much, change as you expected, there are a number of factors that you might examine as a means of troubleshooting the problem. Begin by *asking the patient* what he sees as the problem or barrier to change and whether he has ideas about what could be done to overcome the problem. Frequently the patient will know what to do. If so, reinforce his problem solving and then set a definite time for a reappraisal. Telephone contact can be very useful and reinforcing if you are not seeing the patient frequently.

In other instances the patient will be "stuck," or seem to have no idea what is getting in the way. In this case, begin by exploring whether a behavior incompatible with the plan is being reinforced by another person, or by a consequence you have not thought of. It is often difficult to change behavior without the cooperation of spouses, parents, or other family members.

For example, a dieter may be continually pressured by a spouse to attend dinner parties or to eat forbidden foods. This problem is not easily solved, but sometimes the situation may be restructured so that significant others attempt to help and not hinder the behavior change. A weekend for two or an item each really desires may be negotiated into the contract.

In another example, a child may keep crying and misbehaving in the operatory even though the hygienist reinforces cooperative behavior with attention and "TLC." The misbehavior continues because the parents or siblings continue to give the child attention for it outside of the office. In such a situation you might use one of several different strategies to eliminate or minimize the interfering behavior. For example, you may want to structure time for the child, requiring only five minutes of cooperation to earn a play period or a specific material reinforcer. You might want to work with the parents, instructing them on how to behave appropriately, or even invite them into the operatory. Alternatively, you may decide to use the strategy of extinction and simply ignore the inappropriate behavior of the child.

Check reinforcement procedures:

The problem may lie in the infrequency of the behavior you wish to increase and reinforce. Often the most difficult part of establishing a new habit is remembering to do it! You may find the behavior you wish to change occurs at such a low rate that there are not many opportunities to reinforce it.

Next, check the counting and reinforcement procedures that are being used to make sure that you or your patient are accurately counting and reinforcing the behavior you are trying to modify. Questions that you might ask yourself include:

- Am I reasonably sure that the person is recording the behavior as it occurs, and not just estimating its frequency at the end of each day or week? People who estimate are often tempted to discontinue a plan even though it is succeeding, simply because they believe it is failing. The reverse may also occur, and an ineffective plan may be continued for an inordinate period of time.
- Is the person receiving the reinforcement immediately after he exhibits the appropriate behavior? Timing is important. It is vital in some cases that reinforcement be provided as soon as possible. This is especially true when you are attempting to vary strong habits. For example, biting your nails, smoking a cigarette, or eating chocolate now feels better than the thought of enhancing your health or the prospect of a material reinforcer you will receive next week. By arranging an immediate reinforcement, you can tip the balance toward choice of long-term goals. Praising the smoker when he resists the temptation to light up or the dieter when he turns on the TV after leaving the table without eating seconds is an example.

Reexamine the rewards:

Another common problem involves the nature of the reinforcers. Most of us are not accustomed to rewarding ourselves or others and initially may opt for only modest reinforcement. Discuss with the individual whether he feels the reinforcers are strong enough to help change his behavior. Do they really matter enough for him to make the effort to change?

It is very likely that the consequences you are providing for the performance of the behavior are simply not significant enough. An extra dessert or half an hour of TV time is probably not a strong enough reward to facilitate the patient reaching her objectives. However, something that she considers a luxury will often do the trick. Beefing up the reinforcement can make a real difference. At times, we have found that encouraging a patient to make a down payment or purchase an item on layaway is a useful strategy.

Modify expectations:

Finally, people often design reward systems on an all-or-nothing basis. In such cases, the person has to perform perfectly to receive any reward at all. There is no room for occasional backsliding or nonperformance. Whenever the professional's or the patient's own expectations are too demanding, either for level of performance or rate of progress, failure and discouragement usually follow.

If an initial low frequency of behavior seems to be the problem, there are two things you can do to increase the behavior. (1) Focus on a strategy for actively prompting the individual to perform the behavior. For example, a parent might tell his child when it is appropriate to brush, and then reinforce the behavior immediately after it occurs. Similarly, one might use the alarm on a watch as a cue to monitor posture, or to note jaw clenching. (2) Increase the likelihood that the behavior will occur by pinpointing a behavior closely related to the one you wish to alter but which precedes, or occurs more frequently than, the behavior you wish to modify. For example, if an adolescent washes his hair each morning, you could link that behavior with the less frequently performed behavior of flossing. Begin at a lower level of performance than the one you eventually desire. In other words, "shape" the behavior. Along with failing to provide strong enough reinforcers, one of the most common reasons for failure in behavior change projects is choosing goals and steps that are too big to accomplish.

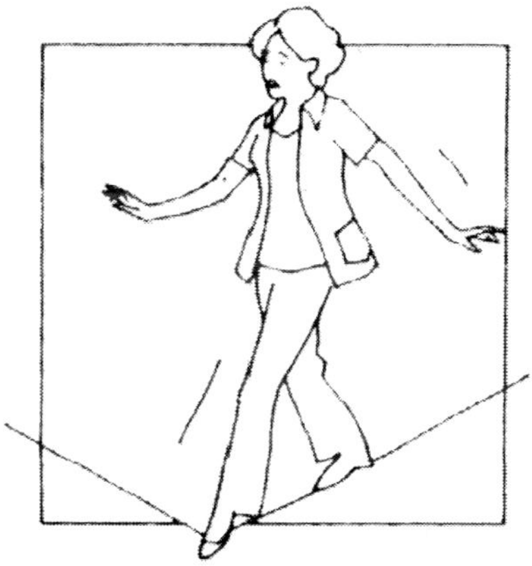

Summary

As problem situations arise, either from your perspective or the patient's, you can rework and modify points of agreement together to help reach objectives. A contract is not an ironclad document. As a health professional, your role is to assist in some way to help change a patient's behavior. It is not to make the patient go along with a given plan. Your flexibility and ability to modify the project will likely be an important factor in its success.

"Great works are performed not by strength, but by perseverance.

S. Johnson"

Chapter 10

Maintaining Change

The final step of the behavior change process typically occurs after a person has maintained the change for sixth months, at which time we say she has moved from the *action* phase to the *maintenance* phase. It is tempting to consider the job done by this time. However, the maintenance phase poses its own unique challenges. For example, individuals who actively work toward weight loss have continual reinforcement through seeing the numbers on the scale drop, but they may find it difficult to maintain that weight loss once they reach their goal weight and once the previous reinforcement no longer exists.

Eliminating the Reward System

As the program progresses and the behavior slowly changes toward the ultimate objective or goal, you must begin to think about eliminating the active intervention phase of the project. If you have used rewards, the first step in this procedure is *phasing out* and eventually eliminating the external reward system. As you recall, when the change procedure is first initiated, some kind of reinforcement should follow every time the desired behavior occurs. As the behavior becomes more established, reinforcement should be thinned out. This process can be accomplished in several ways.

For example, you might increase the level of performance required to obtain the reinforcement. That is, you might start requiring 100 per cent performance or nonperformance, or you might set up a schedule in which you receive a reward only one time in three. In this case you would not reinforce every third occurrence of the behavior but instead would scatter reinforcement in an unpredictable fashion to average one for every third occurrence. In this way, the behavior becomes less and less contingent on a reward.

Eliminating Support Systems

Concurrently with thinning out the reinforcement, give the individual increased responsibility to monitor or administer the program herself. For a young child, this might mean posting her own gold star on the toothbrushing chart. For an adult, it might mean assuming control of a reward system that was originally handled by a spouse, or decreasing the number of checking or monitoring appointments at the dental office. You must be careful to establish this new behavior as firmly as possible in the daily routine of the individual. Remember, the goal is self-maintenance and continuance of the behavior into the future, long after the formal change project ceases.

Follow-up

Once all external monitoring and reinforcements are eliminated, it is easy to find ourselves thinking that the new behavior is established, that we can ease off, and that the change will somehow maintain itself. After all, we wanted change in the first place, and now that we are performing the behavior regularly, why should it fade? Why should we revert to our old pattern? The fact is that new forms of behavior, no matter how enthusiastic or pleased we are with the results, are only tentatively established. It is unlikely that any new behavior or habit will become second nature, especially if that behavior, like all preventive health habits, has no continuing, immediate payoff. There is no immediate consequence for failing to exercise today, or eating two pieces of apple pie, or not

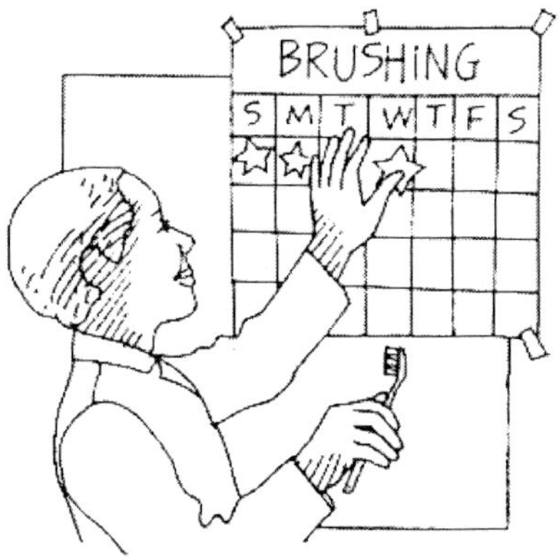

flossing your teeth. Hence, it is critical that some kind of follow-up be established once the project terminates.

One very simple and useful kind of follow-up is self-monitoring. People often find it is useful to continue recording the frequency of the new behavior even though they are no longer receiving any external positive rewards. This recording helps maintain a focus on the new behavior and the changes that have occurred.

Thus, a person who engaged in a weight-loss program might continue to weigh in on a daily or weekly basis, or a smoker might continue to mark "X" in red on the calendar each day he or she succeeds in not smoking.

As we mentioned earlier when we discussed the Premack Principle, or "Grandma's Law," one of the most effective ways to establish a new behavior is to link it to an already well-established behavior. The well-established habit and the use of continued recording serve as cues to help maintain the new behavior.

Another kind of follow-up involves professional monitoring. Recall appointments often function as an important "landmark" or "booster" for patients who need structure and accountability.

Preventing Patient Relapse

There is increasing interest in understanding factors that influence maintenance. Typically, dental professionals' response to difficulties in maintenance has been to increase the number of preventive sessions over a longer period of time. Such approaches have not worked.

We need to understand what influences the *maintenance of* new behaviors. A helpful model has been developed from research in the field of addictive behaviors. This model focuses is on the determinants of recidivism — the tendency to relapse into a previous condition or mode of behavior. Rather than focusing on the question of how initial preventive procedures can be made more effective, the emphasis is on the study of conditions under which prevention does or does not fail, especially the point at which the maintenance of new behavior gives way to backsliding. The rationale for the process of relapse is straightforward. By obtaining information about relapse, you can derive prin-

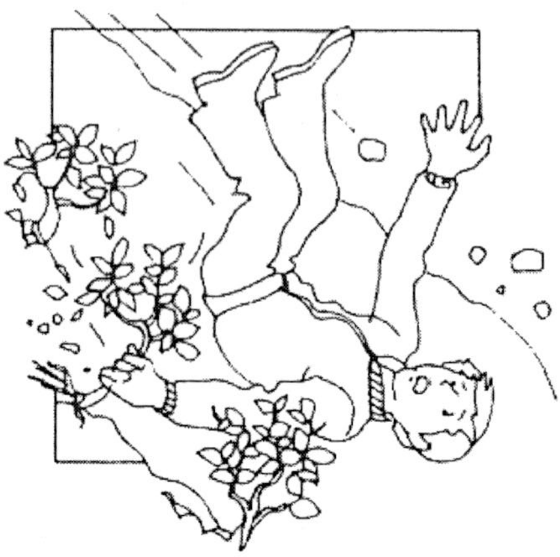

ciples to use in minimizing or preventing its occurrence.

In order to understand the implications of relapse for prevention-oriented programs, a conceptual overview is important. The traditional definition of relapse is a return to a disease state, as in a relapse of malaria symptoms or a fall "off the wagon" after drinking or smoking cessation. Relapse in this definition refers to any return to the former behavior pattern and implies an out-of control state. An alternative viewpoint is reflected in the second definition of "relapse" in Webster's dictionary: "the act or instance of backsliding, worsening, or subsiding." From this perspective, relapse can be viewed as a *single act* of falling back. A more appropriate word we will use to refer to a single occurrence of the specific behavior will be "lapse," defined in Webster's as "an error or slip ... a temporary fall, especially from a higher to lower state."

In the relapse prevention model developed for addictive behaviors, a lapse is viewed as a normal transitional process, a series of events that may or may not be followed by relapse. This concept can be applied in dentistry. Six weeks or so after plaque control instruction, lapses are likely. Life events cause changes in routines that make it more difficult to maintain a high level of oral self-care. From time to time, most of us allow an event (travel, divorce, household move, camping trip, etc.) to influence our self-care habits. Most of us slip from time to time. Whether or not such a lapse leads to a breakdown of the gains made in a plaque control program depends to a large extent on our expectations.

Lapse Versus Relapse

Some individuals do not perceive differences between *lapse* and *relapse*. For them, a single lapse is enough to destroy all of the gains from plaque control. For others, lapses are not significant; they are seen as normal. The psychological literature on relapse suggests that we can reduce the possibility that a lapse will snowball into total relapse. *Most preventive programs are deficient in that they fail to anticipate and plan for the possibility of relapse.* It is almost as if discussing relapse is tantamount to giving the patient permission to relapse. *We believe lapse and relapse should be briefly discussed with patients.* We can "inoculate" our patients against total relapse by giving the patient "permission" to lapse.

Tell your patients that lapsing almost always occurs, but it does not mean they have failed; while it is okay to lapse, it is not okay to relapse. Some lapsing or backsliding is to be expected, but it does not mean that all their effort was for naught. Emphasize to your patients that when it happens—and for most of us it will—they will now have the basic tools and know techniques to implement change. Consequently, they can apply these tools to reestablish the "lost" behavior; it is possible to regain control. Tell patients that a lapse is similar to an error when we are first learning something; we may learn from it. You may also stress that a lapse is usually a unique event.

Relapse Contract

In addition to discussing relapse with patients, a few other strategies are useful. Preventive therapists may wish to set up a "relapse contract" with some patients. Basically this is an agreement concerning the steps to be taken in the event of a relapse. In essence, this agreement reinforces commitment to change and may lead to valuable discussion with patients who express ambivalence regarding maintaining change or who have relapsed in the past. The contract specifies exact procedures to be followed when the patient relapses. Similarly, the "response cost" of an initial slip can be increased by having the patient visit with the preventive therapist, with its associated financial and time costs. Relapse debriefing (an in-depth explanation of what happened) with the therapist is always a good idea.

Programmed relapse is a technique useful when patients do not believe they can make the change last. Agreeing not to clean for a week and to be examined and to debrief afterwards may be a useful strategy. Here, the patient maintains a sense of control and has a heightened sense of awareness of how her mouth feels. Often during relapse a patient will "tune out" her mouth, a reminder of her inadequacy or failure.

Relapse prevention is in its infancy. Expect new strategies to be developed and tested. Most relapse research is being pursued with addictive behaviors. However, problems maintaining positive behaviors such as exercising are also prompting investigators to work in this area.

We have developed a brief relapse questionnaire, shown at the end of this chapter, which can be used to help explore the potential problems of maintenance as the behavior-change program begins to wind down. It can be given in written form, or serve as the basis of an interview-discussion with the patient. The purpose is to solve problems before they actually develop. It may be useful to give this questionnaire at three months to six months after the behavior is established (or eliminated).

Recall: The Booster Session

Another strategy frequently attempted involves the use of a recall, or "booster" sessions, in which the dental professional meets with the patient at various intervals following initial behavior change intervention. The purpose is to bolster and reinforce the effects of the instruction. Research literature in dentistry, medicine, and psychology contains many examples of the effectiveness of the booster strategy.

Twice-a-year patient recall has been a hallmark of contemporary dentistry; however, many patients with a history of significant periodontal disease are recalled more frequently. More frequent recall appointments are particularly useful for patients who have made a significant change in their oral health care habits. Though this is a radical change in protocol, we believe the initial recall session should occur between 30 and 60 days after initial treatment. Although the primary purpose of these visits is periodontal maintenance, they are also excellent opportunities to boost plaque control.

Boosts at recall visits should have two components—*reinstruction* and *motivation*. After the oral examination, provide specific feedback and praise whatever the patient is doing well: "Tell me again why you are trying to ____. Great! Overall, you are doing a good job of cleaning. Tell me, are you having any problems in cleaning? I'd like you to pay special attention to your back teeth, especially the molars on your lower left side. If you can clean this area better, and keep it clean, it could eliminate any need for periodontal surgery. I remember that this is your goal." As you can see, we not only reinstruct, but we also attempt to motivate and, if necessary, to problem solve. If Mrs. Johnson does not routinely use floss, suggest alternatives, e.g., toothpicks. Perhaps her goals were too difficult and she frustrated herself (that is, she lapsed and took the opportunity to relapse). If so, consider renegotiating realistic self-care goals.

As previously noted, it is crucial during these booster sessions to actively question the patient about what problems he sees, what goals he has, and what resistances he may feel. With each new goal will come a different stage of change. Previous successful behavior change will increase a patient's sense of self-confidence and make additional changes easier, but it is important during the booster sessions to assess a patient's readiness to make additional changes. Discuss these changes and remember to reinforce changes that have already been made. Making a significant change and maintaining it for six months is a great accomplishment!

What is the optimal frequency of booster sessions? The patient's level of health, goals, and previous progress are important considerations. As patients show that they are maintaining plaque control, lengthen the intervals—for example, from 3 months to 6 months, or from 6 months to 9 months—with some savings in cost and convenience for the patient. This plan assumes that disease is controlled, and therefore, frequent prophylaxis or periodontal maintenance should not be needed.

For a patient who has relapsed, intervals should be drastically shortened so that she may receive more professional attention and more frequent maintenance. For this unconventional strategy to be effective, the patient must appreciate that to maintain her health, *someone* must remove her plaque. If *she* does the work, she saves money and time. If she does not do the work and is unwilling to pay for services, her health will suffer and the money and time she has already invested in her mouth may be wasted.

What is the best recall mechanism? Some research indicates that a combination of telephone and mailed reminder cards work best (Cohen, Weinstein, and Wurster, 1978). Here is our idea of an efficient recall system: During initial treatment planning, inform the patient that recall appointments are part of his therapy. At the end of a given session, make an appointment for the next. Give the patient a card with not only the date and time of the appointment, but with a detail or two of what will occur at that appointment. For example, we would note that at Mike Johnson's next appointment we will recheck the tooth that received root canal treatment and the areas he had difficulty cleaning.

Some patients are then asked to confirm the appointment in advance by phone or email. Such a request reinforces the active role of the patient in treatment. If he does not call within two weeks of the appointment, a mailed reminder, again with specific details of what is to be accomplished, is sent. Telephone calls are made only to those who do not respond to the mailed reminder. Such a system maximizes recall and minimizes time spent by office staff.

Good communication is extremely important when you are arranging recall appointments. Patients who feel "railroaded" cancel or fail to appear. These patients often perceive recall as an unnecessary expense.

Two studies (Iwata & Becksfort, 1981; Weinstein & Fiset, 1983), found that fee reductions are useful in motivating patients. Both studies refunded part of the professional fee when patients met their prearranged goals of improvement in plaque scores. Such schemes encourage patient recall. In addition, or as an alternative, it is possible to use improved plaque scores as a rationale for less frequent recall. Written agreements or contracts are useful in a rebate scheme to encourage maintenance. Such documents, which should be simply written and signed by dentist and patient, avoid misunderstanding and facilitate performance.

Perspective: Integrating Behavior Change into Your Office

At this point we have covered the seven fundamental steps involved in initiating a change program. By participating in a change project, you experience the different phases of the program and become aware of the difficulties and advantages involved in each step. Moreover, from your own experience in managing change, you become familiar with the difficulties inherent in changing someone else's behavior.

In your own practice, you may not have the opportunity to go through each step with every patient who desires change. However, you now possess a basic understanding of the process that occurs when a person tries to alter his or her behavior. Drawing from this understanding, you should be able to choose the particular sequence of steps or techniques most appropriate to each individual patient.

We do not recommend that you immediately eliminate your present preventive program and substitute our procedures. Rather, it is best, especially while you are gaining experience with behavior change strategies, to use them as a supplement. We will feel that we have succeeded if you have increased your repertoire of techniques for dealing with patients. Practicing these techniques is extremely important. Try them out first on yourself and then on the patients with whom you feel most comfortable.

We hope you will use these techniques in your practice and recommend them as part of a preventive treatment and recall program. It is our experience that patients who successfully change their behavior are the most likely to elect comprehensive care and return for regular recall visits. In addition, the opportunity to work with a patient as much as is required to accomplish behavior change builds rapport and long-term commitment to your practice.

In our own practice, we often charge professional fees for oral hygiene instruction (American Dental Association code 1330) based on the time involved. This is particularly true for initial sessions. In later stages, we include the fee in the charges for prophylaxis (ADA CDT code 1110). A survey we conducted of practices in Washington State found that most practitioners include plaque control fees in the fee for oral hygiene. Nonetheless, we found a trend, especially among periodontists, to charge separately for the service. This trend allows the patient to see these services as distinct and valuable and allows you, the practitioner, to receive a fair return on your professional efforts.

As with any other procedure or program you employ, remember to approach the patient confidently. Your expectations are always perceived by the patient and will influence whether she will be successful in changing her behavior. Aside from the techniques and strategies we have stressed, your enthusiasm and encouragement are the most important factors in helping your patients change their oral habits.

Dentistry, like medicine, has traditionally been disease oriented. Yet practitioners have always recognized that the primary focus on health care should be prevention rather than cure. Louis Pasteur said, "When investigating a disease, I never think of finding a remedy for it, but instead a means of preventing it."

Review of the Behavior Change Process

First Session: Steps 1 and 2

Tasks:

1. Identify the problem to be addressed. Ask questions, listen, and encourage self-motivating statements. Determine the patient's readiness to change a specific behavior.
2. If the patient desires change, determine what instruction the patient may need. Could he make the change if his life depended on it? If "No," instruct before proceeding.
3. Discuss the importance of finding out when and where the behavior is occurring and not occurring. Arrange for the patient to collect baseline data. A contract may be helpful in making the agreement to collect baseline data in preparation for behavior change.

The first step consists of identifying a problem that the patient desires to work on and defining, as specifically as possible, the problem and its probable cause. In other words, what and why. Here we determine if the problem is a skill or a management deficiency. Could the patient brush or floss properly if he or she had to do it? This is also where, through open-ended questions, you assess the patient's readiness to change.

The second step is identifying when and where the behavior occurs or does not occur. Prior to attempting to initiate any change, we must find out specific instances of when and where the behavior is occurring and not occurring. For example, a patient who is in college may or may not be aware that she almost never brushes her teeth on weekends or when she has an early morning class. Information on when and where is usually obtained when baseline data are collected and reviewed by the patient and health professional.

Second Session:

Steps 3 and 4 (about two weeks later)

Tasks:

1. Review the baseline data with patient. Assess and problem solve any resistance to collecting the baseline data. Encourage self-motivating statements.
2. Set overall goals and realistic and specific intermediate objectives. Assess and resolve resistance to goals, and actively involve the patient in goal setting.
3. Plan a strong intervention with input from the patient that uses a number of strategies.
4. Include all relevant information in a contract. Have patient sign it and possibly make it public.

Step 3 consists of examining the baseline data collected by the patient and negotiating overall goals and realistic intermediate objectives that can be reached. Instead of requesting patients to brush and floss more often or better, it is more effective to negotiate a specific and realistic number of times per week as an intermediate objective. For example, a patient who brushes twice a week may be successful in increasing her brushing to four times a week. Requesting her to brush and floss every day may be too high a goal to strive for initially and would result in feelings of failure, as opposed to the feeling of success in meeting a more modest goal.

Step 4 involves problem solving, planning and implementing an intervention method. This phase includes deciding with the patient what will actually be done by both you and the patient to help change the behavior, the results you hope to achieve, and the step-by-step procedure to be followed. To increase your chances of bringing about some positive movement and change, bring more than one intervention strategy to bear on the problem, if possible. Once you have agreed on the specific goals, objectives, and interventions, draw up a contract to be signed by both you and the patient. Remember, the patient must play an active role. Menus and choices are best.

Third Session:
Step 5 (generally 2 weeks to a month later)

Tasks:

1. Review the data collected and charted by the patient. Review any difficulties the patient may have had. Encourage self-motivating statements (for example, ask "Why are you doing this?").
2. Modify the intervention plan and/or objectives, as needed.
3. Rewrite the contract to reflect changes.

Step 5 consists of reviewing and modifying the intervention plan through the remaining phases of the behavior-change process. Review data collected and charted by the patient. In doing so, you will become aware of what seems to be going right and what is not working. It is very common for the initial design to have unforeseen weaknesses. More likely than not, some problems will arise. Encourage the patient to think of the "big picture." Troubleshoot and modify the intervention plan and/or intermediate objectives or even the goals. Revise or rewrite the contract to reflect these changes.

Fourth Session:
Step 6 (generally 2 weeks to a month later)

Tasks:

1. Review the data collected and charted by the patient. Again, encourage the patient to verbalize goals.
2. Plan for self-maintenance and short- and long-term follow-up.

Step 6 involves terminating the formal change project. Every project has a beginning and an end. The end must be as carefully planned as the beginning to avoid backsliding. As careful as you may be in planning and implementing change in habits and behavior, many patients find themselves falling back into old habits and patterns of behavior. Such backsliding should be expected, and plans should be made to minimize its effect. Failure to plan may result in the undoing of all change and could make renewed efforts at changing behavior more difficult. This step consists of formulating and implementing a self-maintenance plan and plans for short- and long-term follow-up visits and/or telephone calls. Remember to encourage self-motivating statements.

Structured Relapse Questionnaire

1. Some people work out specific methods or "tricks" that they feel help them maintain their new habits. Describe the methods or tricks that help you.
2. Have there been any specific situations or events that almost or actually "got in the way" or interfered with maintaining your new habit?
3. Have you experienced any changes in how you feel about or view yourself as a result of your new habit? If yes, describe them.
4. I would like you to indicate how confident you are that you will maintain your new habit at your current or higher

level using a scale of 1 to 10, where 1 indicated low confidence and 10 indicates high confidence.

5. Now that you have been performing your new habit for a while, if you should "slip" for a short period (up to a week), what you do think your chances are of resuming your new habit? Choose a number from 1 to 10, where 1 indicates that such a slip would not affect resuming the new habit and 10 indicates that it would most likely lead to giving up on the new habit entirely.
6. Some people view starting a new habit or stopping an old one as mostly a matter of "will power," while others see it mostly as a matter of replacing one set of habits with another one. On a scale of 1 to 10, where 1 indicates that changing is very much a matter of "will power" and 10 indicates that changing is very much a matter of replacing one habit with another, indicate which best describes how you feel about changing habits.
7. Many people who begin a new habit (for example, quitting smoking or starting a diet) feel that if they have that "first cigarette" or eat a forbidden food just once, they have "blown it" and their efforts to change have failed. Others seem to feel that one cigarette or piece of pie is not very critical and that it was merely a slip. Which do you feel applies to you?
   a. When I have a slip, I am likely to say, "The heck with it" and go back to my old habit(s).
   b. When I slip, I figure that I won't let it get in my way.

Part III:

Special Clinical Problems

"To cease smoking is the easiest thing I ever did. I ought to know because I've done it a thousand times.

M. Twain"

Chapter 11

Tobacco Use —Helping Patients Quit

Knowledge of the health risks of tobacco use is widespread. Yet, as is well known, smoking tobacco (including cigarettes and cigars) has been linked to illnesses that include coronary artery disease, hypertension, and stroke. Tobacco use has also been implicated in oral health conditions that include periodontal disease and oral and throat cancers. Many health organizations, including the American Dental Association and the American Medical Association, have strongly urged health professionals to encourage their patients to stop smoking.

Prevalence of Tobacco Use

Recent estimates suggest that approximately 25 percent of men and 20 percent of women in the United States smoke cigarettes. Tobacco is consumed in several other forms as well, and each carries its own specific health risks.

Smokeless Tobacco

Some people use smokeless ("spit") tobacco products, believing that these products are safe alternatives to smoking cigarettes or cigars. Smokeless tobacco products may be classified into three primary groups:

1. **Chew** – these shredded tobacco leaves are placed as a "wad" between the cheek and gum.
2. **Plug** – similar to chew, shredded tobacco leaves are pressed into a hard block and then placed between the cheek and gum.
3. **Snuff** – this form of tobacco is placed between the gum and bottom lip and consists of ground-up, moist tobacco. This type of tobacco use is known as "dipping."

Rather than being inhaled through a cigarette, nicotine in smokeless tobacco enters the bloodstream more slowly through the oral mucosa, but remains in the bloodstream longer than if inhaled through a cigarette. Smokeless tobacco users, therefore, may become addicted to nicotine more quickly than smokers. In addition to nicotine, smokeless tobacco products contain other substances that may negatively affect oral health. Abrasives found on tobacco leaves can wear down tooth surfaces, and sweeteners, which contribute to tooth decay, are often added to tobacco to improve its taste.

Despite its reputation as a "safe alternative" to smoking cigarettes, smokeless tobacco poses many of the same health risks as smoking cigarettes, as well as additional health dangers. Use of smokeless tobacco has been linked to heart disease, oral and throat cancers, stomach ulcers and cancer, and various oral conditions such as periodontal disease, tooth decay, and stained teeth. Because of these health risks, the American Dental Association has officially stated its opposition to the use of smokeless tobacco as a smoking cessation method.

Why Don't People Just Quit?

In light of the many health risks associated with all forms of tobacco use, it may be difficult for many health professionals to understand why their patients continue to use tobacco products. The following are factors that may contribute to sustained tobacco use:

Nicotine Addiction

Nicotine has been shown to be a highly addictive substance, sometimes described as more addictive than even cocaine or heroin. Research has suggested that nicotine strongly affects receptors in the brain, altering brain chemistry and causing a strong positive feeling, or "euphoria." It is, in part, this euphoric feeling that reinforces people for smoking or using smokeless tobacco.

Behavioral Aspects

Very often, the use of tobacco products is strongly associated with pleasurable activities. For example, many smokers have cigarettes with their morning coffee or when taking a break from work. When attempting to quit, smokers need to break themselves not just of the habit of smoking, but also of the connection between smoking and pleasurable activities.

Social Factors

Many individuals who use tobacco products do so with other people. For example, we have all seen groups of people smoking outside of public buildings because they are not allowed to smoke inside. Taking a "cigarette break" allows people to socialize and take a scheduled time away from their work. Many people report that they feel "left out" of social situations once they quit smoking, because they are no longer spending as much time with their friends and co-workers who continue to smoke. In addition, some individuals' spouses or partners continue to smoke after they have quit, making it more likely that those who have quit will be tempted to start smoking again.

Environmental Cues

Reminders in the environment may make smoking cessation difficult. Even though cigarette advertisements are now more strictly regulated, objects such as ashtrays, lighters, and matchbooks can serve as cues to encourage people to smoke, particularly if they are trying to quit. As many people try to quit by "just not thinking about smoking," these environmental cues make abstaining from smoking even more difficult.

Discussing Quitting with Patients

Smokers are constantly reminded that they should stop smoking. Health care professionals, friends, family members, and the media provide consistent messages that smoking is harmful. Warnings about smokeless tobacco are less common but are becoming more prevalent as more is learned about the health risks associated with this form of tobacco. As previously discussed, however, many factors that contribute to use of tobacco products are not addressed by "just saying no" or lecturing patients about the harmful effects of tobacco.

It takes more than health professionals' advice for patients to stop using tobacco products. As described in earlier chapters, dental professionals are in a unique position to assess patients' motivation to change their behaviors by asking supportive, open-ended questions. Parker (2003) specifically describes ways in which dental hygienists may address smoking cessation with their patients. Koerber and colleagues (2003) showed that dental students receiving brief training in Motivational Interviewing (MI) for smoking cessation were able to engage patients in discussions of smoking cessation significantly more than students not trained in MI.

Just as it is important to assess patients' readiness to change their oral self-care, so is it important to understand their readiness to stop using tobacco products. The methods described in the Motivational Interviewing chapter to assess patients' readiness for change can be used to understand what motivates each individual to use tobacco and what motivates him or her to stop using tobacco. Specifically, it is crucial to assess both how *willing* and how *able* patients are to stop using tobacco.

When a patient is responding to your questions, demonstrate listening without judgment (as described in the Motivational Interviewing chapter). Don't argue with the patient, even if you don't agree with his statements. Use empathic statements to let him know you understand the difficulty of quitting tobacco use, even though he knows tobacco use is harmful.

Patient: I've tried to quit a million times before, but just can't stick with it.

Dental Professional: It sounds like you've made a lot of great attempts to stop in the past, but some things have gotten in the way of stopping for good.

Patient: Yeah, something always comes up that gets me started again.

Dental Professional: What kinds of things have come up in the past?

Patient: You know, life in general. I stopped a few years back, and then my son dropped out of school and I got really stressed out. Then there was another time when, the day after I quit, I got laid off from work. I figured, what the heck? I might as well smoke; I have nothing better to do.

Dental Professional: So, smoking helps you feel less stressed out.

Patient: Definitely. I mean, I know it only makes things worse, but I can't help it, you know?

Dental Professional: Sure. In the short term, it makes you feel better, but in the long term…?

Patient: I always feel like I blew it, and that just makes me feel more stressed out.

Dental Professional: Well, you've already made some great attempts at quitting, and we know that most people need to try to stop more than once before they quit for good. Would it be okay if we talked a little more about ways to improve your chances for success if you try again?

Did you know? Most people quit smoking several times before they stop for good. Research shows that every time people try to quit smoking, they learn new strategies for remaining tobacco-free. After two or three (on average) quit attempts, people have enough "tricks" for quitting to allow them to stop using tobacco permanently. Patients who relapse after quitting smoking should be encouraged to continue their efforts to remain tobacco-free and learn from their previous lapses (and/or relapses) to help them succeed on their next attempts to quit.

Expressing understanding and empathy to a patient lets her know you're concerned about her health without lecturing her. Nearly every patient will express ambivalence toward quitting tobacco and will likely express concern about her ability to quit. Again, arguing against ambivalence will likely cause the patient to argue with *you* and be less likely to want to make a change. However, helping her to verbalize benefits of quitting and her barriers to change will allow you to work together to problem solve in each situation. The primary goals of the dental professional, then, are to help patients identify possible barriers to change and provide them with tools to overcome these barriers.

Below are some "dos" and "don'ts" for assessing a patient's readiness for change:

- **DO** ask the patient what he enjoys about using tobacco, as well as what he does not enjoy. In other words, ask about the pros and cons of using tobacco.
- **DO** ask him about pros and cons of *quitting* tobacco.
- **DO** listen attentively. Maintain direct eye contact and make sure you're paying full attention to him. Ask questions as needed to clarify what he is saying. (For example, "So, what I hear you saying is that you want to stop smoking, but have had trouble in the past?")
- **DO** rephrase a patient's statements, but **DON'T** repeat them back word for word. For example, if he says, "I just can't quit smoking!" Don't repeat back, "You can't quit smoking." Instead, say, "Trying to quit smoking has been a tough journey for you so far."
- **DO** demonstrate understanding. Nod when appropriate, but not excessively. Rephrase the patient's statements as appropriate.
- **DO** use "I statements," such as "I'd like to spend a little time talking to you about smoking, because I'm concerned about

how it might affect your teeth."

- **DON'T** use "you statements," such as "You need to stop smoking because you're putting your life in danger."
- **DON'T** argue with a patient. For example, if she says, "All my friends from work smoke," do not argue "They're making the same mistake that you are!"
- **DON'T** rush the discussion. If you don't have time on one particular day to discuss tobacco cessation, ask the patient, "Would it be okay if we talked more about smoking the next time you come in?"
- **DON'T** use "scare tactics." For example, don't tell a patient, "If you don't stop smoking, you'll get oral cancer and all of your teeth will fall out from periodontal disease. Is that what you want?"
- **DON'T** dismiss the patient if she isn't ready to discuss tobacco cessation (e.g., "Hey, it's your life, I don't care what you do.") You can always leave the door open by saying, "So, what I hear you saying is that right now isn't a great time for you to stop smoking. Would it be okay with you if I check back with you about it the next time you're in?"

Tools to Help Patients Quit

Once patients have expressed willingness to stop smoking or using smokeless tobacco, dental professionals are in a unique position to provide many different tools to help achieve this goal. We can help each patient develop a "game plan" for quitting. This can include behavioral changes, pharmacological methods, or a combination of both.

Behavioral Changes

When patients are preparing to stop using tobacco, dental professionals have many behavioral tools to offer. The more "tools in the toolbox" you are able to provide for patients, the more likely they are to succeed.

1. **Identify triggers** – As previously discussed, tobacco use is often closely associated with everyday activities and emotions. Encourage patients to identify what triggers them to smoke or chew tobacco so that they are able to plan ahead for times when they are most likely to want to use tobacco. Some examples are:
    - after meals
    - when waking up in the morning or just before bed
    - taking a break from work
    - drinking alcohol or coffee
    - feeling lonely, stressed, or angry
    - driving
    - watching TV
    - being with other smokers or seeing others smoke

A patient may keep a "smoking log" for a week or two prior to quitting, in which he records when he used tobacco (day and time), where he smoked or chewed (in the car, at work), and how he is feeling (stressed, angry, sad). This will him identify when he is most likely to want to use tobacco.

2. **Planning for trigger situations** – Once a patient has identified situations during which she is most likely to want to use tobacco, ask her to identify other activities she might be able to do in these situations to avoid smoking. Planning ahead for trigger situations helps patients feel more "in control" of quitting, and decreases the chances of relapse. For example:

- Encourage a patient to do other things with his hands when he would typically smoke. Holding pens, water bottles, paper clips, and other objects will help distract him from not holding a cigarette.
- A patient may chew sugarless gum, suck lollipops or mints, or eat carrots or celery sticks so that she has something in her mouth. She should also be encouraged to brush her teeth immediately after meals

so that she is not tempted to use tobacco after she eats.

- Encourage the patient to avoid situations with other smokers, at least when he is first quitting. If he goes to restaurants that allow smoking, he should sit in non-smoking sections. He can also spend more time with his non-smoking friends and family members.
- A patient should avoid or cut down on alcohol use, as this can be a strong trigger for smoking or chewing and can impede his judgment and motivation to abstain from tobacco.

Let patients know they will probably not need to give up certain activities forever, but simply to avoid them when they are first abstaining from tobacco use. For example, a patient will not have to cut ties with her friends who smoke, but should probably spend less time with these friends until she feels more confident in her ability to abstain from tobacco while in the presence of other smokers.

3. **Plan a specific quit date** – All the experts agree that it is important to decide on a specific date to quit. This date should be far enough in the future to give the patient time to prepare to quit, but not so far in advance that he can easily "push off" or delay it. Planning this date around a significant milestone may help him stay focused. For example, he may want to quit smoking before a family member's wedding, before he buys a new car, or before Christmas. Of course, a quit date should not occur at the same time as a potentially stressful situation (a friend's surgery, a stressful family gathering, a significant meeting at work, etc.). Stressful situations can often sabotage a successful plan to quit.
4. **Tell others about the quit date** – Many people do not want to tell others that they are planning to quit (so that they will not be embarrassed if they are not successful). However, telling friends, co-workers, and family members about the quit date helps a patient build a support

network. In this way, he has many people encouraging him and helping him stay focused on his goals.

5. **Plan to stay busy –** In addition to planning for specific trigger situations, encourage patients to plan enjoyable activities to help them stay busy. Walking, playing tennis or golf, riding a bicycle, going to the movies or mall, or playing with children or pets can help people distract themselves from the desire to use tobacco.

6. **Plan short- and long-term rewards –** Encourage patients to notice positive physical signs while they are abstaining from tobacco, such as breathing more easily and being able to do more physical activity with less difficulty. Also encourage them to reward themselves for remaining abstinent from tobacco. Some short-term rewards (i.e., for one day, a week, two weeks without tobacco) may be:

   - A new music CD
   - A new book by a favorite author
   - A new pair of shoes or piece of clothing
   - Taking a long walk in a favorite area
   - Taking time to read the newspaper or a magazine

   Long-term rewards should be more extravagant than short-term rewards, but still fit within reasonable time and financial limits. Long-term rewards may be planned for remaining tobacco-free for one month, six months, a year, or more, and can include:

   - A weekend trip to a new or favorite spot
   - A new outfit, or several new pieces of clothing
   - A trip to a day spa

7. **Anticipate brief lapses –** As explained in the chapter on motivational interviewing, many people will have "slips" while they are trying to abstain from tobacco. It is important for a patient to acknowledge these "slips," or "lapses," and understand what caused them. (Was she

under an unusual amount of stress? Was she in a situation with a lot of smokers?). It is also important for dental professionals to let the patient know that slips are normal and not a sign that she will not be able to quit successfully. Many people feel that if they have even one cigarette or one bit of smokeless tobacco, they have "blown" their chances to quit and will resume using tobacco as they had before. Patients should not be reprimanded for slips, but instead should be encouraged to immediately "get back on the horse" and resume their efforts to avoid tobacco. It is important to remind patients to not let a slip or lapse become a relapse.

8. **Practice makes perfect** – Many people require more than one attempt before they successfully quit smoking for good. People learn from their previous mistakes each time they attempt to stop using tobacco, and their chances of stopping tobacco use permanently increase with each quit attempt. Remind patients that both persistence and planning pay off when trying to stop using tobacco.

It should be noted that many health insurance companies offer low-cost or free smoking cessation counseling programs and usually offer reduced premiums for non-smokers. Dental professionals can advise patients of these health insurance benefits as further encouragement to stop using tobacco.

Medications to Help Patients Quit

For many people, pharmacological methods can help make avoiding tobacco easier and increase success of long-term abstinence from tobacco. As with any medication, of course, it is very important to consider possible contraindications for specific patients prior to suggesting pharmacological methods for tobacco cessation. However, many people benefit from the use of nicotine replacement therapies and report fewer withdrawal symptoms with their use. Usually, these medications are used by heavy smokers.

- **Bupropion** – Marketed under the brand names "Wellbutrin" and "Zyban," bupropion is usually prescribed in pill form to be begun one week prior to the quit date. The primary role of bupropion is to help alleviate withdrawal symptoms. It is also marketed as an anti-depressant but does not seem to have different effects on tobacco cessation between patients with and without a history of depression. Patients with a history of seizures or eating disorders, or who are already taking anti-depressant medications, should not take bupropion.
- **Nicotine gum** – Although this product is referred to as "gum," patients should be instructed to hold this material between the cheek and gum to release nicotine into the bloodstream through the mucosa instead of chewing the material. They should also be instructed to not smoke cigarettes or use smokeless tobacco at the same time they are using the nicotine gum, as this will lead to large amounts of nicotine being released into the bloodstream.
- **Nicotine lozenge** – Similar to nicotine gum, the lozenge is held in the mouth and allowed to dissolve while the nicotine is absorbed through the oral mucosa. Possible side effects include sore throat, tooth and gum sensitivity, and indigestion. These symptoms typically diminish with time and use of the product. Patients should be advised not to bite or chew the lozenge, as this will result in a large dose of nicotine being absorbed at once.
- **Nicotine patch** – The nicotine patch works similarly to a self-adhesive bandage and releases a constant amount of nicotine into the bloodstream through the skin. Patients are instructed to wear the patch 24 hours per day to avoid nicotine withdrawal symptoms. Sleep disturbance and skin rashes may develop as a result of using the patch, and patients should be advised not to smoke or use smokeless tobacco while using the patch. This prevents releases of large doses of nicotine into the bloodstream.

- **Nicotine inhaler** – Also called a "puffer," this thin cartridge resembles a cigarette. It allows patients to "puff" without inhaling the same level of nicotine and other harmful substances that they would with a cigarette. Nicotine is contained in a capsule at the bottom of the inhaler and is delivered into the bloodstream through the oral mucosa as the patient inhales through the cartridge. Patients may experience irritation of the lining of the mouth, coughing, runny nose, and indigestion. These symptoms tend to diminish with time and product use.
- **Nicotine nasal spray** – This product is usually recommended for patients who are highly dependent on nicotine, as the nicotine is absorbed through the nasal mucosa and provides a faster "hit" than other means. Compared with other nicotine replacement methods, the nasal spray allows patients to control the doses of nicotine they receive. Common side effects include irritation of the nose and throat, which tend to diminish with time and product use.

As with all medications, patients should be instructed to carefully follow all instructions provided with nicotine replacement methods and should consult with a health professional prior to beginning or changing any medication regimen.

Combining Methods to Quit

Smoking cessation research generally suggests that individuals are more successful in stopping tobacco use when they combine nicotine replacement medications with behavioral methods for abstaining from tobacco. For example, a patient who uses a nicotine patch should still set a quit date, tell others around him that he plans to quit, and establish a plan for coping with trigger situations. Similarly, another patient who uses bupropion should avoid situations in which others are smoking, and she should set up short- and long-term rewards for avoiding tobacco. However, patients should not combine two or more nicotine replacement methods, and they should always consult a health professional prior to beginning or changing pharmacological methods for tobacco cessation.

Dental professionals, then, are in a unique position to assess patients' readiness to begin a tobacco cessation program, educate them about various behavioral and pharmacological methods to quit, and encourage them to remain abstinent from tobacco products. Quite possibly, the most important role dental professionals play in tobacco cessation programs is to follow up with patients, encouraging them to avoid tobacco and educating them about improvements seen in their oral health as a result of tobacco cessation.

Finally, below we list some additional references that dental professionals may use to help their patients stop using tobacco products. Many of these references include information for health professionals as well as for patients.

- U.S. Department of Health & Human Services, 2000. *Treating Tobacco Use and Dependence: A Public Health Service Clinical Practice Guideline*. http://www.ahrq.gov/path/tobacco.htm
- National Cancer Institute, 1994. *Tobacco and the Clinician: Interventions for Medical and Dental Practice*. Monograph #5 of Smoking and Tobacco Control Monographs. (The entire monograph or selected chapters may be downloaded from http://cancercontrol.cancer.gov/tcrb/monographs/5/index.html).
- Society for Research on Nicotine and Tobacco, 2003. *Treatobacco.net: Database & Educational Resource for Treatment of Tobacco Dependence*. http://www.treatobacco.net/home/home.cfm

You can also recommend the following resources to your patients:

- Centers for Disease Control, 2005: The online version of the "You Can Quit Smoking" Consumer Guide: http://www.cdc.gov/tobacco/quit/canquit.htm

- Smokefree.gov, 2003. *Clearing the Air.* http://www.smokefree.gov/. This Web site is a joint effort of the Centers for Disease Control, National Cancer Institute, and American Cancer Society. This site has resources for people trying to quit as well as health professionals.
- Boston University School of Public Health, 1995: http://www.quitnet.com/

Assignment for Chapter 11

OBSERVER CHECKLIST

____ Uses open-ended questions

How many?____________

____ Uses reflective listening

____ Simple reflections

____ Amplified reflections

____ Double-sided reflections

____ Gives advice suggestions

____ Reassures

____ Interrupts, asks questions, changes topic

____ Judgmental expression

Comments:______________________________

The following exercises are designed to be done first as a classroom activity, then with a patient you identify in your practice. These exercises are similar to the activities discussed in the Motivational Interviewing chapter, and specifically address smoking cessation. The exercises below involve groups of three. Each learner will practice and receive feedback. If time permits play all three persons: speaker, listener, and observer. The following form is useful in providing feedback:

> When doing these exercises in class, if you are the individual acting as the smoker but you do not smoke, think of reasons for smoking that you have heard from people who do smoke.

Assignment 1:

Person 1 will tell Person 2 about a habit that he or she has tried to stop in the past without success (for example, nailbiting, snacking between meals, etc).

Person 1 will reveal the information reluctantly and slowly.

Person 2 will use as many reflective listening techniques as possible. (Please see the Motivational Interviewing chapter for a review of these skills.)

Person 3 will give feedback to Person 2. Person 1 will also comment on the interview.

Assignment 2:

Person 1 is a new patient who smokes a pack and a half per day.

Person 2, as the dental provider, will try to establish rapport and trust and then ask about the patient's feelings about quitting smoking. Person 1 should express *willingness* to quit.

Person 2 should be sure to address the following issues:

- Assess the patient's readiness to change. What stage of change is the patient in? What reason(s) do you have to think this?
- What barriers to quitting does the patient face?
- What benefits does the patient see in quitting?
- Do the barriers outweigh the benefits, or vice versa?
- What can Person 2 say to Person 1 to move him/her farther along the stage of change? For example, are there behavioral or pharmacological aids you can offer?

Person 3 will give feedback to Person 2. Person 1 will also comment on the interview.

Assignment 3

Person 1 is a new patient who smokes a pack and a half per day.

Person 2, as the dental provider, will try to establish rapport and trust and then ask about the patient's feelings about quitting smoking. Person 1 should express *resistance* to quitting.

Person 2 should be sure to cover the same issues as described in Assignment 2.

At the end of the dialogue, all members of the group should discuss the differences between working with a patient who is willing to change versus one who is resistant to change. How do you change your approach between these two types of patients?

Assignment 4

If possible, identify a friend, family member, or patient who currently smokes and would be willing to discuss quitting smoking with you. Be sure to address the same issues with this person as described above (i.e., readiness to quit, barriers, benefits, resistance), and follow the steps you have learned to move her/him further along in the stages of change. Be sure to help the person set realistic goals. For example, if your subject currently smokes one pack a day, a realistic goal may be to cut out 1 or 2 cigarettes per day for a week, then 1 or 2 more cigarettes per day the following week.

“The obscure we see eventually. The completely obvious, it seems, takes longer.”

E. R. Murrow

Chapter 12

Oral Self Care and Children

Many health professionals are reluctant to treat children because they fear difficult management problems. In many instances a lack of adequate training and experience may increase the problem, and result in the attitude that these patients are not worth the effort. Although the principles and strategies we have discussed in the previous chapters are effective for patients of all ages, we have added a chapter to examine special considerations for children. This is precisely because practitioners often find that children present special problems in communication. Further, the goals for treating children often differ from the goals for treating adults.

Child Dental Fear

Dental fears begin in childhood. Creating positive attitudes in children toward dental care might therefore be the most effective strategy to create positive attitudes toward dentistry in the population at large. For children, early dental experiences must occur with a minimum of physical and psychological trauma.

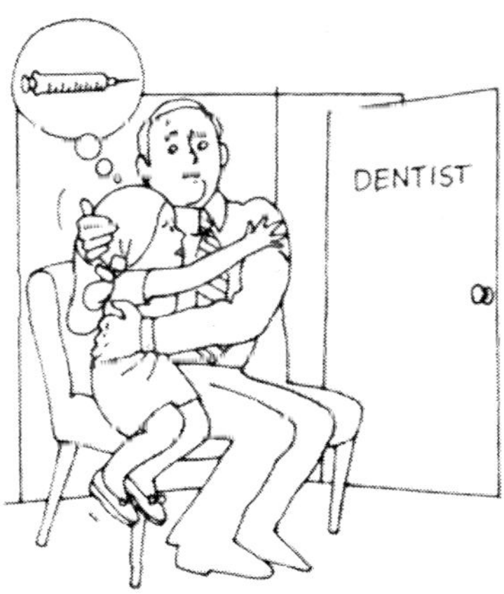

The child's behavior is the most important factor affecting actual treatment. Without a patient's cooperation, all dental procedures become difficult; thus the need for effective, humane behavior management of children is obvious.

We have learned that the effect of a traumatic dental visit may be influenced by previous dental experiences. The greater the number of positive experiences, the greater the likelihood that when a "bad experience" occurs, it will not lead to severe fear or phobia. Fostering a positive, trauma-free dental history should be the goal of every clinician who interacts with children.

The child who becomes very fearful after a trauma (and successfully avoids dental care afterwards) is usually the one with a limited history of preventive care. Usually he or she visits the dentist only to have problems diagnosed and teeth restored or extracted. Such episodic care is scary; something is done to you with sharp instruments after you are separated from your mom or dad. Preventive care, on the other hand, allows more participation by the child (and parent). Although it may require considerable cooperation, e.g., placement of sealants, it minimizes trauma. Further, such care has the obvious benefit of reducing the need for restorative dental services.

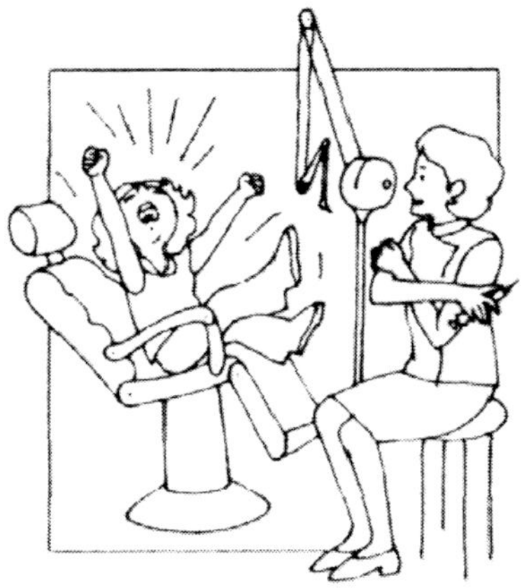

In order to promote humane treatment and lifelong acceptance of dental care, we recommend that practitioners attempt to create an accepting, "safe," child-oriented environment, a place for the child to explore and learn. We want the child to learn that the dental office is not scary and that he or she has the opportunity to learn to cope with dental procedures. In doing so, we recognize that children are different from adults and that developmental factors are at work.

Feeling trapped and vulnerable contributes to fear. Even though parents and their surrogates, including dentists, need to maintain ultimate responsibility, they can help the child exercise some degree of control over events. A safe environment is one in which the child actively participates to some extent and *feels* he or she is in control. Children who believe the environment is responsive to their desires show less fear. More about this important topic is presented in our text *Treating Fearful Dental Patients.*

How to Deal with Parents

Highly anxious parents tend to have uncooperative children. Interestingly, researchers have found that when anxious mothers attempt to reduce their children's anxieties, they paradoxically increase anxiety. Apparently some mothers (and fathers) do not know how to prepare their children for dental visits. One practical approach to this problem involves sending a pre-appointment letter to parents of each new child patient. The letter should be something like this:

YOUR CHILD'S FIRST DENTAL VISIT

Dear Mrs./Mr. ______________,

I am writing to you to thank you for the interest you are showing in your child's dental health by making an appointment for a dental examination. Children who have their first dental exam when they are very young are likely to see dental care as positive throughout life.

At our first appointment, we will examine your child's teeth and gums and maybe take x rays. For most children this proves to be an interesting and even fun time. All of the people on our staff enjoy children and know how to work with them.

Parents play an important role in getting children started with a good attitude toward dental care, and your cooperation is much appreciated. One of the useful things you can do is to be natural and easygoing when you tell your child about his appointment. This will allow him to view his appointment as a chance to meet some new people who are excited to meet him and want to help him stay healthy.

Good general health depends in large part upon good habits, such as good eating and sleeping, exercise, and fun activities. Dental health also depends on good habits, including proper toothbrushing, regular visits to the dentist, and avoiding too many sweets. We will have a chance to discuss these points further when you come to the office.

Best wishes, and I look forward to seeing you.

Sincerely,

One last issue, which has been the focus of countless discussions and papers, is whether you should allow the parent in the operatory. Although the experts tend to disagree, we believe the mother or father should be allowed to remain in the operatory 1) if the parent is not overtly anxious, and 2) as long as the parent does not interfere with treatment. It is important to tell the parent the ground rules, i.e., that you are the expert and he or she must respond, even if he or she does not at the moment personally agree with your approach. At times, especially with young children, the parent may be helpful in reducing anxiety and increasing cooperation. Her presence also may avoid the compounding effect of traumatic separation. However, there are times when the child will show less cooperation when the parent is present.

Parents or other responsible members of the family must be present when we are focusing on oral self-care. They will be the child's oral care

Child Oral Self Care Activities

Children learn to stand, walk, talk, sing, and play. More importantly to us as health professionals, they learn at an early age a variety of hygiene skills essential in our society. Behavioral techniques have been extremely successful in helping normal children master toilet training without trauma. Therefore, it is not surprising that behavioral techniques have been used in teaching oral hygiene skills to children.

The Preschool Child

Child tooth cleaning

Should a young child be given a toothbrush? Anxious parents often question us about instructing their two-and-a-half-year-old to clean her teeth. We believe that young children can begin to take some responsibility for their oral health. Tooth cleaning should be encouraged as another activity the child can begin to master.

We counsel parents to slowly shape the tooth cleaning behavior of the child and to be patient and accepting of his low level of fine motor skill. The initial goal should be to familiarize him with tooth cleaning tools and sensations; this should always be fun. Although his dexterity may be minimal, the child is beginning to develop a habit that will last a lifetime. The effectiveness of his cleaning should not be of concern. Let him practice as you observe him. Provide plenty of positive social reinforcement.

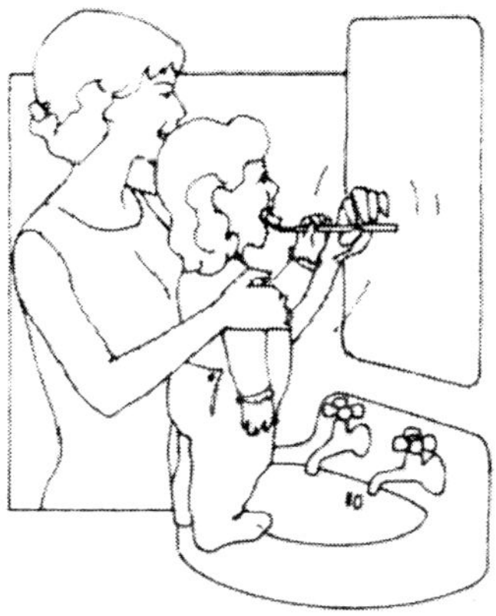

Parental tooth cleaning

The parent should be instructed to clean even the young child's teeth once a day, preferably after the child has completed her "cleaning." Parents should receive a formal lesson in cleaning their children's teeth. Supervised practice is always necessary when these skills are being learned. Although there are many ways to position oneself when cleaning a child's teeth, we recommend you try this: have the child stand directly in front of you, both facing the mirror. Place your cheek against hers and begin to clean. This may be easier than facing the child and trying to view her teeth while cleaning. Remember, the child, though relatively passive, still needs considerable positive reinforcement.

While many children enjoy the soothing sensation that a toothbrush provides when massaging teeth and gingiva, some children resist when a parent or another attempts to clean. When a parent tells us that they face stiff resistance from their child, we usually follow the protocol below:

Resistant child protocol

Motivate the parent

- Ask what the parent does to keep the child safe in a motor vehicle. Discuss child resistance and parental response to resistance.
- Ask about parents' or family's dental health. What would they want for their child? Rate the importance (See the Motivational Interviewing chapter earlier in this book).
- Tell the parent you have worked with parents who have had similar problems and ask whether or not they would like to learn about how other parents like themselves solved this problem. Ask the parent if she is willing to try an experiment.

Locate time and place

- Encourage the parent to choose a quiet time in a comfortable room (not necessarily the bathroom). Many parents choose the bedroom at bedtime.

Use gradual exposure, a behavioral approach

The procedure described below is effective if entered into with a spirit of playfulness. Grim determination is not helpful, as a resistant child will mirror the parent's feelings. It seems to be best to make a game of it.

- Introduce the brush. Give the child a brush (with no dentifrice) to hold. See if the child places the brush in his mouth—a good sign.
- "Take turns." Take out *another* brush and place it in *your* mouth.

- Ask the child to brush *your* teeth for a count of five, using fingers to keep track of time.
- Tell the child it is now *his turn.* Brush his teeth to a count of five. Continue taking turns. (Cue the parent to tell the child how much she appreciates his cooperation. Verbal reinforcement, hugs, and kisses are very appropriate.)
- Introduce dentifrice. Put a little on your finger and run your finger across your own teeth. Mmm! Now on the child's finger. If the child does not want to put his finger with the dentifrice on it into his mouth, be silly; encourage the child to put the dentifrice on his nose (or even on your nose first!).
- Put toothpaste on the brush. Take turns. Ask the child to put the brush with dentifrice in your mouth. If you feel like it, cooperate minimally by moving your head or not opening your lips very wide at first. Say "Now it is your turn!" Count to five or ten and then stop for a treat or a rest or play break. Stretch the brushing time by telling an interesting story while your child brushes.

What to do when the child strongly resists

Again, counsel the parent not to show upset or impatience. Break the problem into smaller pieces. Encourage making a game of it.

- The first time or first few times, play with your toothbrush by yourself with the child watching. Brush your finger, then your arm, and then your cheek. Increase the amount of time, slowly. Total time should not be over 2–3 minutes. This should be done prior to sleep or at another comfortable time.
- After the child has watched you for a few nights, give *her* a turn. This should be fun, with hugs and kisses and verbal reinforcement.
- Over time, place the brush to the child's lips, then in her mouth. Model the behavior on yourself, too.

Once the brush is in your child's mouth, with you holding it, ask her if she wants to hold it too. Move the brush for a count of five, ten, etc.

Keep it short. Take turns, especially if the child likes to take turns.

A very small percentage of children will not allow others to touch them without significant protest. Autistic children and children with a history of post-traumatic stress are more likely to present this problem. Parents of very resistant children need much encouragement. It may be useful to schedule frequent, brief sessions to work with parent and child. If this is not feasible, try frequent telephone contacts to reinforce the parents' enthusiasm and to problem solve.

This approach is useful for typical children as well as those with special needs. It clearly relies on parental competence and patience. If parents are not comfortable with this role, ask if they have a relative or friend who could work with the child.

Verbal reinforcement, hugs, and kisses should always be part of teaching children. Material reinforcement and tokens can also be very useful. This book's chapters on behavioral technology contain many suggestions about how to use reinforcement.

The School Age Child

As the level of dexterity permits, a parent or other adult can give the child a lesson in tooth cleaning with a toothbrush. This should involve demonstration and supervised practice with much praise and small material rewards. Parents should observe the child and should be told to watch the child clean at home for at least several months.

Parents ore caretakers should identify a time and a place to do a thorough cleaning. Some families are strapped for time in the morning. They should be encouraged to make their efforts in the evening, as part of a nighttime family ritual. We recommend that parents use the Premack Principle, doing the thorough cleaning before another regular activity, such as bathing.

The good taste and sensations of tooth cleaning offer some intrinsic reinforcement. However, it is extrinsic reinforcement that may help the child go through the effort needed to establish a relatively difficult new behavior. In addition to social reinforcement, which should always be provided profusely, and a minimum of criticism or negative social reinforcement, material and activity reinforcers may be employed successfully with children.

We often recommend that dental personnel help parents negotiate an agreement with their child. The agreement, which may be written in contract form, specifies the rewards a child will receive for his or her tooth cleaning activities. Amount and kind of reinforcers should be noted. Bonus clauses for sustained or exceptional performance are also possibilities. Remember, no legal jargon; this is simply a clear agreement between people specifying how they will behave toward one another. An example of such an agreement between parent and child is presented here.

In addition, many benefits are gained from using monitoring charts. Children may place stars or stickers on a calendar for every day they clean their teeth, as agreed to in their contract, or they may color the calendar. Moreover, the child can make his own calendar. Such charts not only cue behavior but they rewarding in and of themselves. Remember to recommend that the child change the chart regularly. Children become bored with sameness.

Tooth Cleaning Agreement

(Mom) and (Patty) agree to work together to help keep Patty's teeth healthy and beautiful.

What the child (Patty) agrees to do:

- *Try to remember to clean my teeth at least once a day just like the dental hygienist (Mary) showed me and (my Mom).*
- *Ask (Mom) to check out my teeth when I finish.*
- *Put a star on my chart every day I clean like I was shown.*

What the parent (Mom) agrees to do:

- *Remind (Patty) to clean at the regular time and place.*
- *Avoid nagging when (Patty) does not clean; at that time clean her teeth for her.*
- *After she is finished, tell (Patty) how happy I am to have her clean her own teeth.*

- *Check (Patty's) teeth (once) a week with the "magic pink pill" that turns plaque, tongue, and lips red.*
- *Give out gold stars to be placed on the chart—(one) gold star(s) for each self-cleaning, (two) gold star(s) for a good job when the magic pink pill is used.*

What the child (Patty) will get:

- *(Mom) agrees to (read you a story) right after (every time) she gives you a star.*
- *When you have earned (five) stars, she will (buy you the toy you really want).*

What (Mom) will get:

- *(Patty) will have clean teeth and fewer cavities.*
- *Fewer arguments and whining.*

(Mom) signature ________________________________

(Patty) signature ________________________________

Note: *Signatures are optional, and should be used only if they are not seen as coercive by the patient.*

The Adolescent Child

Adolescents often complain they do not receive enough information and they are not given meaningful choices. They are often told what to do, at times without a compelling explanation. All of us have a desire to establish and maintain our independence of action, and this motivation is particularly strong in adolescents. Adolescents often respond poorly to being told what to do—even when they know what they are being told to do is in their best interest. This is called *reactance.*

Because of reactance, adolescents are perhaps the most difficult to work with. Moreover, they are neither children nor adults. Often they talk to us like adults but may respond like children. Much patience and tolerance are required. Moreover, adolescents frequently do not perceive the worth of the preventive measures we expect them to perform. We explain why they should do something and then let them go off on their own. Later, they are often chided for not meeting our expectations. Because they are sensitive to criticism, such feedback often results in conflict or avoidance.

Getting input from the adolescent is often a useful strategy. What is the adolescent's internal motivation to clean his teeth? What does he want from his mouth? From his dentist? Hygienist? Base rate measures are often useful, for they focus attention without criticism and allow the adolescent to change "by himself." In addition, it is often useful to ask adolescents what it will take to help them clean effectively. Would checking in with someone be useful? Structure may be useful, especially if *they* tell you so. How about rewards? Cleaning is hard work. The message we want to give you is that you should fully explore "doing it their way."

Hygienist: Nate, I want to talk to you about how you look at your teeth and mouth.

Nate: Okay, sure

Hygienist: Some teens are really very concerned about how their teeth look. Others don't care very much at all. Some teens are concerned about their breath, not wanting to offend others or be rejected or put down. Some teens just want to minimize hassles in their life—for example, to find the simplest way to keep others off their back about how they take care of themselves. Tell me what you are concerned about?

Nate: I'm more of a keep-them-off-my-back sort of guy.

Hygienist: Okay, this is important to know. If you are interested, I am willing to talk to you about what other teens have done to keep people from getting on their case.

Nate: Okay, I'm all ears.

Hygienist: First of all, the teens were willing to gather accurate information about how they clean their teeth and the amount of time/effort it takes. If I have this information, I can problem solve with you to find the quickest and easiest way for you, maybe even with a bit of hands-on help from me on a regular basis, to keep your teeth from being a problem that would lead others to dump on you.

Other behavioral techniques are also useful. Contracting, especially for activities and social rewards, may help. However, the clinician should tell the adolescent of her willingness to modify the agreement and even to write this into the contract. Modest goals and small steps are still needed for these older children. One last word of advice: be sure to let them know it's okay to miss a day or even a week of cleaning. Not only will you guard against relapse, your permission to slip will guard against some forms of adolescent rebellion or "testing the limits."

"Motivation is the art of getting people to do what you want them to do because they want to do it.

D. D. Eisenhower"

Chapter 13

Working with Orthodontic Patients

Concerns about "White Spots" Post-Treatment

Orthodontists and staff members in orthodontic practices often are concerned about the potential for lawsuits and malpractice claims over "white spots" or cavities in the front teeth that are detected after orthodontic appliances are removed. Such patients also may have red and bleeding gums during treatment because their hygiene is so poor. In one study Gorelick and colleagues (1982) found that 50 percent of patients in fixed appliances had at least one "white spot" by the end of treatment. Another study found similar results (Ogaard, 1989).

The usual response to this clinical problem is *reactive*. That is, we try to motivate these patients—usually teens—to improve their home care. We give them bags of special brushes, Superfloss®, floss threaders, and disclosing tablets with the hope that things will improve; and things often do get better for a while, with hygiene regressing to baseline soon thereafter. As clinicians, we get frustrated, plead and cajole, and eventually we bring in the parents as the "big guns" to try to gain improved cooperation. When this fails, in the worse cases the braces are removed and a structured dismissal plan is implemented (Machen, 1990).

Our goal in this chapter is to identify skills that clinicians can use to prevent "white spots" and cavities and therefore angry or dissatisfied parents at the finish of treatment.

In this chapter we argue for a *proactive* approach to the inevitable difficulties that child and teen patients face in adapting to orthodontic appliances. As with the other problems, we see a return to good oral health as the sum of activities by the patient and the professional. When the patient does less than is needed, the professional picks up the slack. The mutually agreed upon goal is good health, and the implicit contract recognizes that at various times the patient and clinician will be able to assume different levels of responsibility. This approach builds trust and rapport and avoids staff burnout. Imagine this conversation:

Orthodontic Preventive Assistant: Jason, next week Dr. Good Good will be putting on your braces. Are you excited about it?

Jason: Yeah, I guess so...

Assistant: You don't seem that enthusiastic.

Jason: Well my mom really wants me to do this...

Assistant: I'm glad you told me this.

Jason: Yeah, some of my friends tell me it's a pain to brush your teeth with the braces. The orthodontist and their parents are always on them about this.

Assistant: Sounds like you don't want the hassles of braces that are being forced on you by your mom.

Jason: You got it.

Assistant: I'd like to help you minimize the hassles, if you are interested. I will show you the easiest way to clean your teeth, and when you come in I promise not to get on your case about how you're doing. I'll offer things for you to try and I'll try to do things here to make it easier.

This kind of conversation is a tip-off that your goals for this teenager's home care should be initially very limited. You'll need to do more to keep him healthy. The intent is to take small steps to gain cooperation and to identify internal motivation. In this kind of relationship, external motivation is less effective. Teenagers always have a choice not to cooperate, and they can get pretty stubborn in the short run even if the result is not in their best interest in the long run. Rapport and trust are essential in any professional relationship, especially with older children and teens. If we find ourselves pleading and then threatening a child, we know its time to take a step back and reassess the situation. Something is not working.

Stages of Change

In this chapter we will discuss both behavioral and chemotherapeutic approaches and how to put them together for the benefit of orthodontic patients. First, let's review what we learned earlier about stages of change. The idea is that not all of our patients are ready to adopt the new and cumbersome oral hygiene behaviors required of an orthodontic patient. Many times the motivation for seeking orthodontic treatment is from the parents. They are thinking about the long-term welfare of their child and are willing to bear the time and financial costs of several years of treatment. The role of the child in this decision-making is secondary. In some cases the child may have been given few options. Thus, it is possible that your young patient may be in the *precontemplative* stage. He or she may not have considered the benefits or problems of treatment and may not be ready to assume much responsibility. Imagine the following conversation:

Bill: My parents are just pushing this whole braces thing on me.

Assistant: I get it; nobody really listened to what you thought about the whole thing?

Bill: Yeah.

Assistant: While I am not in a position to tell your parents not to go ahead with your braces, tell me about your concerns about braces.

Bill: It seems like a major pain, and I'm okay with how I look.

Assistant: Much effort with no payoff? Tell me about the positives and negatives of braces for you.

Bill: I'll have to miss band practice. I'll have to wear dorky, uncomfortable headgear. And my mom is on my case about keeping my teeth clean, even before I've got the braces on!

Assistant: Wow, plenty of negatives. Any positives?

Bill: For my parents—they want my teeth to look better and they insist on braces NOW.

Assistant: You seem annoyed at your parents forcing you into braces, but it seems like you do what your parents tell you to do.

Bill: I guess so.

Assistant: Well, it seems to me that at best, you are concerned about the negatives.

Bill: Yes I am.

Assistant: Bill, my experience is that you may find it helpful to learn a little bit about how others who didn't want to have braces have managed with braces on. Would you be interested in hearing about the experiences of other guys like yourself and how they minimized the hassles?

Bill may be reluctant, but the idea is to begin slowly. It is like the old saw about the encyclopedia salesman getting his foot in the door. You need to start somewhere in order to make a sale. In working with orthodontic patients you face the same problem. To move from *precontemplative* to *contemplative* is a big step. All the while you substitute therapeutic alternatives to try to keep Bill healthy. The rate of change from one stage to the other, *contemplative* to *action* for example, will vary between patients. When you know you have the alternatives to offer that will allow the patient to be healthy in spite of lack of optimal home care, you don't have to plead or coerce. Over time, most of your patients will take steps to cooperate further. This avoids professional frustration and burnout.

The Run-In

The second critical strategy in working with orthodontic patients is called the "run-in." The basic idea is to try to improve self-care before placing the appliances, because if it is not good before, it certainly will not improve once the appliances are placed. In the period when records are made and treatment planning is under way, the effort to teach new oral hygiene skills should begin. It is the time, as we have discussed in earlier chapters, to offer choices about how to best maintain oral health and see what options the child and family would like to follow. This is the time for initial skill training in tooth brushing. Recall that many young people spend less time cleaning than optimal and may not be very effective for the time they put in. Since our goal is to prevent damage to the upper anterior teeth, this is the best place to begin. Try to assess whether this patient would have the skill to clean his anterior teeth if his life depended on it or if he is ham-handed. If skill is the problem, and it will often be, start there. Consider using the same type of toothbrush you want the patient to use after the braces are in place. This is also a good time to check out the place where this person will be cleaning. Is there good light? Is there a place to store the cleaning paraphernalia you'll eventually be offering? When are the best times of day to clean?

If the patient has the skills to clean but is slow to adopt the cleaning behaviors you recommend—even before the braces are placed—take a step back and see if you can get him to comply with a simpler, less burdensome request. This is the time also to begin the therapeutic alternatives discussed later in this chapter. Remember the deal you made with Bill—you make up for what he doesn't or can't do, and the sum of the efforts is a healthy patient.

This time before the braces are placed is also a good time for involving the parent. You'll remember from the chapters on behavioral technology that parents can be the source of potent reinforcement for required behaviors. At this stage, and during various rough periods during treatment, the parents will need to take increased responsibility. Some busy parents may be resistant to having to supervise tooth cleaning. That is normal. Imagine this conversation:

Orthodontic Preventive Assistant: Mrs. Garcia, I need you to help us out while Maria gets used to cleaning her teeth with the new braces. In the beginning you'll need to keep a chart of when she cleans and help her use the red disclosing tablets to check how she is doing.

Mrs. Garcia: She can do it herself. She is a good brusher; and besides, I am busy with my job and her younger brother.

Assistant: I hear you. I have a couple of kids at home too. It can be hard. We'll need your help for a short time just to help get things going. In our experience, without your help at this early time Maria will be at risk. Can we have your help on this? I will try to keep it simple. If it doesn't work, we'll change it. OK?

After the Braces Are Placed

This third step is definitely the time to keep it simple. A big bag of cleaning tools may seem like a good idea, but you'll find few patients actually use them. The basic idea is to make a plan and to introduce new cleaning tools only as rapidly as your patient can accept and use them. Remember always that as clinicians we tend to underestimate how hard it is to learn a cleaning skill. Be patient, break the skill up in small steps, and always be positive. If something is not working, try something else. Imagine this conversation:

Orthodontic preventive assistant: Hey, Sally! It's great that you got the braces on your top teeth.

Sally: I don't know. It hurts.

Assistant: You're right, but this stage will pass quickly and you'll like the changes in how your teeth look. I'd like to teach you one or two things that will help you keep yourself more comfortable. OK?

Sally: I guess so...

Assistant: How about if we practice removing some of the bread and other gross gunk that is accumulating around the braces in the front?

Many skilled assistants find that a small tufted brush works well in this situation. However, whatever you choose, have the patient try it, emphasizing the skill part, and find something else if it does not seem to be working. While you're developing these skills, it is time to implement your part of the bargain: the therapeutic alternatives.

Therapeutic Alternatives

Good oral health is always the sum of activities by the patient and the professional. In the previous chapter on therapeutic alternatives, we provided an overview of the basic options a clinician has at his or her disposal. In this section of this chapter we will discuss some of these alternatives from an orthodontic perspective.

Fluoride and Other Strategies

A recent review found that daily 0.05% sodium fluoride rinses had been shown to be fairly effective in preventing the development of "white spots" on teeth during fixed appliance therapy (Benson, Parkin *et al.*, 2004). However, it is important to note that only 13 percent of participants in a key study fully complied with the protocol, and 45 percent used the rinse less than every other day (Geiger, Gorelick *et al.*, 1992). Daily rinsing requires a compliant patient. The alternatives we choose need to require little or no adherence. They need to be professionally delivered. Children and teenagers are likely to come for the adjustments of their braces, so they are readily available for our intervention.

Now let's get back to basics by focusing on the clinician's part in the therapeutic partnership. The same review cited above, which found that rinses were effective, also found some evidence that glass ionomer fluoride-releasing cements (GIC) were helpful in preventing "white spots." A more recent systematic review confirmed the effect. It found that for every five brackets placed with GIC, one cavity would be prevented (Derks, 2004). One of the best studies compared GIC from Dentsply in Germany to no-mix composite resin from Unitek and showed a difference in favor of the glass ionomer (Marcusson, Norevall & Persson, 1997). Many studies of bonding use a small number of subjects or are not of very high quality. Nonetheless, using GIC to bond brackets and bands appears to be a viable step.

As in the case of dental caries in general, regular and high fluoride toothpastes are effective "white spot" preventives. Unfortunately, these strategies have not been well studied in orthodontic patients.

However, there is no reason to believe they would not work. Given that plaque accumulation is greater around brackets and bands than in normal dentition, the use of a triclosan -containing anti plaque toothpaste (for example, Colgate Total®) or a xylitol containing fluoride paste (for example, Crest Multi Care Cool Mint) may be an appropriate strategy. Even though the brushing itself maybe hit and miss, the fluoride plus the triclosan or xylitol will be delivered. It is likely that use of xylitol is more sensitive to how often it is used than is triclosan.

A number of studies compare manual and electric toothbrushes or compare types of both. These studies have mixed results, and differences are likely due to the novelty of electric brushes. Nevertheless, it stands to reason that an electric brush may be helpful to some orthodontic patients who are struggling with a manual brush. Careful attention to design is important. Electric models with a rotary oscillating design appear to work better for patients without appliances (Robinson *et al.*, 2005). Several have been suggested to be effective for orthodontic patients (Heintze *et al.*, 1996; Ho & Niederman, 1997), and differences between them are likely to be a matter of personal preference. Nevertheless, brushes with timers that cue patients are more likely to be effective than those without timers.

Topical fluoride varnish is a well-proven preventive agent. As we discussed earlier, varnish is more effective than fluoride gels. Todd and colleagues (1999) reported a 50-percent reduction of demineralization around brackets in a laboratory study of extracted teeth with an experimental caries challenge. In a patient who is at high risk for caries—one who has had decay before or who has poor hygiene—a varnish treatment at every adjustment appointment is not unreasonable.

Xylitol

Xylitol gum or other xylitol products are excellent vehicles for caries prevention. Often patients who are unwilling to use a toothbrush effectively are willing to chew gum. Regular use of gum (Isotupa *et al.*, 1995; Stecksen-Blicks *et al.*, 2004) and lozenges (Segun *et al.*, 2004) results in reduction of mutans streptococci in plaque around brackets and leads to improvement in recovery from a low-pH challenge.

Xylitol products need to be used at least three times per day and at a minimum of six grams per day to be effective (Ly *et al.*, 2006).

Chlorhexidine

Regular use of chlorhexidine rinses carries with it some of the same pluses and minuses as other strategies for reducing plaque and its consequences, as do fluoride mouth rinses. In addition, some patients experience tooth sensitivity, and others react to the taste of the rinse. Chlorhexidine should be used twice per day at least 65 percent of the week to have much effect. However, if an orthodontic patient tastes it and does not find it objectionable, it may be a viable therapeutic alternative (Anderson, 2003).

Awareness of Interference with Adherence: Developing Sensitivity to Teen Stress and Depression

Teens who are stressed out or depressed are not likely to cooperate with oral self care regimens. Moreover, they are likely to have a variety of problems, from keeping appointments to using headgear. These are the kids who repeatedly bust arch wires.

"Happy Days" images of the teen years frequently underestimate the turmoil felt by teens. Life for many adolescents is difficult, filled with demands from parents, teachers, coaches, employers, peers, and themselves. Growing up—negotiating a path between independence and reliance on adults—is tough and can create lots of stress. Teens can be stressed for a number of reasons: breaking up with boy/girlfriend; arguments or conflicts with parents, siblings or peers; arguments or conflicts between parents; change in familial financial status or address; serious illness or injury of family member or friend; performance in school and elsewhere. For some teens the stresses are too great, and the internal and external resources available to them are limited. Depression is a frequent consequence that can lead to other problems such as eating and sleeping disorders and substance abuse.

How do I know whether or not a teen is stressed out or depressed?

1. Is the teen performing all the normal activities of daily living? For example, is the teen who previously was neat and clean now disheveled and dirty?
2. Is the teen who was doing well in school having academic problems?
3. Is the teen visibly anxious or loudly argumentative and angry?
4. Is the teen disinterested in an activity or sport that was once important?
5. Is the teen "emotional," easily upset?
6. Does the teen ignore parental direction?

Talk to the teen and listen

Ask open-ended questions to establish rapport and trust. "Tell me what you would like to do (if you could)?" is a good question that most teens will answer. That question can be followed by, "Now tell me what you do not like to do? Ask questions about teen culture—favorite music, shows, sports, etc. Demonstrate your listening skills by paraphrasing and summarizing what the teen has said on an ongoing basis.

Treat the teen as an adult

Assume that the teen can choose to participate or not participate in all activities. That is, interact with him as if he were completely independent.

1. Offer as many choices as possible, whenever possible.
2. Provide information in as much detail as appreciated. Teens like to be treated as if they are intelligent. Discuss the advantages/disadvantages of different cleaning approaches; the timing of appointments and the use of

headgear, etc.

3. Talk about a partnership between staff and teen. Two-way communication is very helpful. Encourage the teen to ask questions. This allows you to ask questions of the teen.
4. Avoid threats and dishonesty. It is not the staff's job to coerce the teen to participate (this is the parent's job, and It usually does not work anyway). Dishonesty, whether not telling the truth or omitting information, will result in the end of the partnership.

"How far you go in life depends on your being tender with the young, compassionate with the aged, sympathetic with the striving and tolerant of the weak and strong. Because someday in your life you will have been all of these.

G. W. Carver"

Chapter 14

Adaptive Strategies for Patients with Special Needs and the Elderly

Dental Needs of Patients with Special Needs

Patients with special needs—those with physical and cognitive limitations—are perfect examples of our need to balance self care with professionally delivered therapeutic alternatives. Those patients with good parental support or with conscientious caretakers in institutional settings are best able to practice good assisted oral self-care. Those without such support—likely the major part of this group—will benefit by the professional assuming greater responsibility.

Many vulnerable patients with special needs have multiple unmet needs. Study after study demonstrates this fact and reinforces the need for effective primary prevention beginning with infants and toddlers. Opportunities for such interventions exist in the United States in working with Birth to Three Developmental Centers and what is now called Early Head Start in most communities. Such centers are offered under the U.S. Individuals with Disabilities Education Act and have well-trained staff. Centers may offer developmental screening, evaluation and assessment, occupational and physical therapy, speech-language therapy, oral, motor and feeding therapy, early education and playgroups, and parent education and support. Similar programs exist in other countries.

Any dental office can establish a relationship with a center. Children in these centers need to establish a dental home if the families have not identified one previously. Oftentimes parents and caretakers are overwhelmed by providing for other aspects of the disability and neglect the teeth. Medications, the way children are fed, or diet may exacerbate the problem. By starting early in life, the primary activity required is prevention. Many children with developmental disabilities, such as autistism, benefit from having the same routine every day. Children will gradually get used to performing all the evening activities, including brushing, bath, etc., in the same manner and order.

Steps Worth Taking with Very Young Patients with Special Needs

Work with parents on oral hygiene. Every child needs daily oral hygiene, including fluoridated toothpaste. Oral hygiene needs to start with the eruption of the first tooth. Some parents may have been told to wait to use toothpaste until children are older because of concerns about fluorosis. The benefit of fluoridated toothpaste outweighs the risk of fluorosis. Many of children with disabilities are at risk for massive tooth decay, so every step to prevent disease is worth taking. Parents and caretakers need support in learning to look at and clean their child's teeth.

Start with "Lift the Lip". Initially every parent or caretaker should learn to position a small child and use a toothbrush and/or mouth mirror to examine the teeth. A very young child should be positioned on his back, lying on the laps of adults who are sitting knee to knee, with the child's head in the lap of the parent. Coach the parent on how to look at the teeth by lifting first the upper, then the lower lip to look at the child's teeth. Use photographs to help parents learn how to recognize "white spots" or frank cavitation. Teach parents about tooth development and when they should expect to see the teeth emerge. Urge the parents to seek a dental consultation if they discern problems.

Teach the parent to clean the teeth. It can be a struggle to clean the teeth of a growing toddler. Parents should start with the knee-to-knee position for small children. Coach parents to use the toothbrush to clean all tooth surfaces, again using toothpaste. Special finger brushes or even a washcloth can be helpful. Ask the parents where and how they will clean at home. Reassure parents that the initial resistance of the child will decrease if they practice hygiene every day.

Encourage fluoridated water. It is important to find out the source of water for the child and encourage the use of fluoridated tap water.

Apply fluoride varnish. Children with special needs should receive topical fluoride varnish treatments no less than two to three times per year, according to their risk. It is best to clean the teeth first with a toothbrush or washcloth and then apply the varnish. The knee-to-knee position is easiest if the child is small. More information on fluoride varnish and related interventions can be found in the "Therapeutic Alternatives" chapter.

Steps for Various Special-Needs Patients

Research has amply demonstrated that many patients with special needs can learn to clean their teeth. Some of the basic principles that apply are given in this book's chapters on behavioral technology. Older and younger patients alike may benefit from the use of high-fluoride toothpaste and many of the other strategies discussed in the chapter in this book on Therapeutic Alternatives. A partnership involving parent/caretaker, the patient, and the clinician is always needed to prevent and control disease, especially caries.

Many patients with disabilities suffer from fine and gross motor deficiencies that reduce their ability to brush effectively. A horizontal brushing technique is recommended because of its easiness and capability of yielding good results. Special adaptive cleaning aids—toothbrushes with large handles, for example—are available. Companies such as RADIUS Tooth Brush (www.radiustoothbrush.com) make brushes that are adapted for people who have difficulty grasping a normal brush. For some, an electric toothbrush is helpful. A brush with a timer may help individuals with cognitive deficits remember to brush long enough or to change quadrants. The behavioral technologies discussed in earlier chapters can be used in conjunction with these devices to help individuals and their caretakers adopt new behaviors and maintain them. An efficient plaque control program is important to assess and monitor the level of oral hygiene achieved by people with disabilities. You can use disclosing tablets to demonstrate to parents or caretakers how to clean effectively.

All older patients with special needs who have chronically deficient oral hygiene and high rates of caries should be on regular daily fluoride rinse programs with 0.05% sodium fluoride solution if possible in addition to brushing with fluoride toothpaste. Fluoride rinses are available over the counter, and research demonstrates amply that they prevent tooth decay. Nightly application of a 0.4% stannous fluoride brush-on gel has also proven successful in decreasing dental decay in children. This highly-concentrated fluoride gel is prescribed to the child by a dental professional. Older patients also benefit from topical fluoride varnish treatments at least twice per year or more. Some children with disabilities are at high risk for periodontal disease and gingivitis. Brushing the teeth and gums with a 0.12% chlorhexidine gluconate rinse (available by prescription) is helpful if the child is not able to rinse properly.

As mentioned before, dental care at home should begin in infancy. Resistant infants and toddlers are easily handled by two adults using the above-mentioned knee-to-knee position. Usually the child will get used to the brushing and be less resistant. Many older children with disabilities, however, are unwilling or physically unable to cooperate during the brushing. The parents and guardians of these patients will need some advice on how to position and, if necessary, safely restrain a child during the brushing. There are several positions for toothbrushing that allow adequate visibility, convenient positioning, and firm control for the adult, along with reasonable comfort and support for the child. Parents can attach behavioral rewards, such as songs and riddles, to these brushing times to make the situation special to the child. Here are some examples of commonly used techniques:

- The child is standing or sitting in front of the adult so that the adult can hold his head with one hand while using the other hand to brush.
- The child is sitting in the wheelchair with the adult standing behind. The child's head is angled backwards, resting on the adult's torso. The adult uses one hand to support her head and the other to brush her teeth.
- The child lies on a couch, bed, or floor with his head on the parent's lap. The parent stabilizes the head with one hand while brushing the child's teeth with the other.
- Two adults may be required for brushing the teeth of an extremely difficult child.

Some children have a tendency to bite down very hard when their teeth are brushed, making brushing extremely difficult. Parents can use wrapped tongue blades or an extra toothbrush to hold the mouth open while brushing the teeth on one side of the mouth and then doing the same thing on the opposite side. It is very important to stabilize the child's head when using this technique to prevent any injury from sudden movements.

With this population, as well as the elderly, discussed below, medication use, mental illness, stress, xerostomic (dry mouth), and conditions such as Sjögren's syndrome can reduce salivation and increase the risk of dental caries. Salivary substitutes and mouth wetting agents are available and can be recommended. A useful place to find about these materials is the Sjogren's Foundation website (http://www.sjogrens.org).

Dental Needs of the Elderly

The oral cavity, like other parts of the body, is subject to problems of chronic disease associated with the aging process. The elderly have the greatest oral health needs of any segment of our population. Oral health is particularly problematic for the elderly partially or completely edentulous patient. Dentures are frequently used well beyond their normal life. Many elderly patients do not seek regular treatment that could enable them to maintain mastication and prevent irritation of denture-bearing tissue. As the fit deteriorates, the elderly patient will often select a diet that fails to meet bodily needs, consuming food low in proteins and high in carbohydrates and fats.

Although some problems are a result of the aging process itself, others are related primarily to attitudes toward aging. Many older persons tend to react passively to the effects of aging on both appearance and function. They are also more likely to believe that many preventable losses, illnesses, and pain are an unavoidable part of aging. Consequently, they may have a fatalistic attitude toward their health and may be less likely to take steps to guard their physical wellbeing or be concerned with prevention of disease.

There is a correlation between aging and dental disease, but the relationship is not necessarily causal. Dental educators and researchers are now attempting to foster a rehabilitative-preventive approach to the oral problems of the aged. Problems of diseased and missing teeth, ill-fitting dentures, soft tissue disease, and bone deterioration are amenable to rehabilitation, if not prevention. The consequences of poor oral health in the elderly may lead to inadequate diet and malnutrition, pain, infection, and impaired social functioning.

Providing preventive care to elderly patients is challenging; it is often difficult to motivate them to seek dental care, or to make efforts to correct or prevent problems that they do not believe to be severely handicapping. On the other hand, there is evidence that a behavioral approach can be successfully applied to the elderly in modifying diverse health behaviors.

Steps Worth Taking with Elderly Patients

Establish rapport. Time invested in establishing rapport with older patients is not wasted. You should appear unhurried and take time to chat with the patient. A general suspicion of professionals by many elderly patients warrants your conveying a personal interest in them. Remove your mask and talk face to face. Facial cues provide important cues to comprehension. The natural visual and auditory losses of aging require close interpersonal distances. Avoid physical barriers.

For example, sit next to the patient, not behind a desk. Physical contact can also be reassuring. Providing care for elderly people involves special attention to their physical comfort. Always offer assistance in and out of the chair and cushions for back support.

Gradually introduce into the conversation your questions about previous dental care. The questions may provoke revealing answers. Perhaps the patient is worried about cost or discomfort. Or perhaps he does not really want dental care and came only at the insistence of a relative or friend. Patients' answers to questions about loss of teeth and the wearing of dentures are also helpful in planning future treatment.

Assess psychological factors. Before performing extensive and expensive dental work, conduct an evaluation of the patient's personal values regarding the importance of oral health and her more general approach to life. These are important factors in her satisfaction with your work and may relate to how well she will maintain a prosthetic appliance or a program of oral hygiene. A positive approach to life and people, as opposed to a critical or disturbed approach, is conducive to satisfaction with dental care. Similarly, the perception of the practitioner as helpful and kind is important. The practitioner's best source of data for assessing these factors is the patient's verbal and non-verbal behavior during her interaction with the staff in the dental setting.

Depression is common later in life, affecting more than 6.5 million of the 35 million Americans who are 65 and older. Only about 10 percent receive treatment. Older women are twice as likely to be depressed as older men. Unmarried or widowed people and those with thin or non-existent support systems are at high risk. Depression in the elderly is associated with dependency, chronic illness and disability, and the side effects of medications. It is not an inevitable part of the aging process

Depression itself may have an effect on oral health. Depression is associated with periodontal disease, caries, and myofascial pain and TMJ Disorder. Depressed people do not readily seek out dental services and are not likely to comply fully with recommendations. Minimizing the need for active patient cooperation is essential. Simple treatments that minimize the number of appointments are recommended.

Treat elderly patients with dignity. Many elderly people are sensitive to their perceived loss of status and esteem. Remember that through death of loved ones, loss of work role, lessened financial security, and reduction of physical abilities, many elderly persons lose their own sense of competence and independence. Consequently, it is extremely important to treat the elderly individual with respect. Involve the patient in treatment planning. When you are ready to consult with the patient, move from the operatory to the office. Minimize outside distractions and noise.

Write it down. Give the patient a diagnosis, treatment plan, or other information in writing. Vision, memory, and hearing losses occur frequently, but many elderly patients do not want to admit the deterioration of their faculties. Written information allows the patient to stay in control. Many elderly people are sensitive to their loss of status and esteem; extreme courtesy is always warranted.

Whether or not you use a written plan, you should encourage the elderly patient not to make an immediate decision, especially if feelings about the treatment plan appear uncertain. The patient should have time to think and/or seek the opinion of family, a friend, or other professionals.

Expect active participation. After the patient accepts a treatment plan—for example, when he decides to have a new denture fabricated—it is helpful to involve him in every stage of the process for selecting teeth. By participating in each decision, the patient is less likely to feel "pushed." This involvement will result in fewer complaints, corrective work, and rejections. Similarly, request that your elderly patients maintain their own oral hygiene, as you would do with other patients, and work with them in this effort. Many practitioners inadvertently discourage the self-maintaining behaviors of elderly patients by unburdening them of responsibilities for their own maintenance. Encourage patients to strive for some level of competence and control over their lives. When treated as deficient, most patients will react by meeting your low expectations. Self-fulfilling prophecies occur at all ages.

We find behavior change techniques can be applied to a variety of problematic behavior patterns of elderly persons, although a few minor adjustments may be necessary. There is some evidence that elderly people need more encouragement than younger people. Reinforcement for effort is especially important. Objectives should be relatively short-term and uncomplicated, because long-range, complex plans are especially likely to have a negative influence on the decisions and behavior of many elderly people.

Go slowly. Although aging does not necessarily result in deterioration of mental abilities, elderly people often appreciate having more time to absorb information or make decisions. Their comprehension is as great as that of younger individuals, but they tend to be cautious. They want to be accurate. Take extra time to communicate effectively and do not overload them with information. Give instructions slowly and clearly. Written instructions are an effective follow-up to verbal direction, and written material should be in large, clear letters. When you are speaking with the patient, eliminate extraneous background noises. Stereo systems and even fish tank pumps make hearing more difficult. Careful arrangement of material is also important; the less complex the better.

Limit your expectations concerning what can be mastered at a given appointment. When attempting to learn new skills, such as proper brushing or flossing, everyone's performance usually begins at a low level and increases with practice. Elderly patients need more repetitions and pauses during practice in order to reach the same standards as those reached by younger people. Your creativity may be called into play to find solutions to elderly patients' dental self-care problems caused by limitations in vision or impaired dexterity from arthritis. Electric toothbrushes are very valuable for the elderly whose dexterity is limited.

References

Adams KE. Patient choice of provider gender. *Journal of the American Medical Women's Association*. 2003 Spring; 58:117–9.

American Dental Association (2000). *Summary of Policy and Recommendations Regarding Tobacco*. Retrieved August 22, 2005, from http://www.ada.org/prof/resources/positions/statements/tobac.asp

American Medical Association. Physician Responsibilities for Tobacco Cessation. (*AMA Policy* No. H-490.917). Chicago, IL: Author, 2005.

American Psychiatric Association. *Diagnostic and Statistical Manual of Mental Disorders* (Fourth Edition). Washington, D.C.: American Psychiatric Association Press, 1994.

Anderson MH. A review of the efficacy of chlorhexidine on dental caries and the caries infection. *Journal of the California Dental Association*. 2003 Mar; 31:211–4.

Astroth DB, Cross-Poline GH, Stach DJ, Tilliss TS, Annan SD. *The Transtheoretical Model: An approach to behavior change. Journal of Dental Hygiene*. 2002 Fall; 76:286–95.

Axelsson P, Lindhe J. Efficacy of mouthrinses in inhibiting dental plaque and gingivitis in man. *Journal of Clinical Periodontology*, 1987 Apr; 14:205–12.

Axelsson P, Nystrom B, Lindhe J. The long-term effect of a plaque control program on tooth mortality, caries and periodontal disease in adults. Results after 30 years of maintenance. *Journal of Clinical Periodontology*. 2004 Sept; 31:749–57.

Axelsson P, Paulander J, Nordkvist K, Karlsson R. Effect of fluoride containing dentifrice, mouthrinsing, and varnish on approximal dental caries in a 3-year clinical trial. *Community Dentistry and Oral Epidemiology*. 1987 Aug; 15:177–80.

Benson, PE, Parkin N, Millett DT, Dyer FE, Vine S, Shah A. Fluorides for the prevention of white spots on teeth during fixed brace treatment. *The Cochrane Database of Systematic Reviews 2004* May; Issue 3: Art. No: CD003809.pub2. DOI:10.1002/14651858. CD003809.pub2. Amended 21 May 2004.

Benson PE, Shah AA, Millett DT, Dyer F, Parkin N, Vine RS. Fluorides, orthodontics and demineralization: a systematic review. *Journal of Orthodontics*. 2005 Jun; 32:102–14.

Burke BL, Arkowitz H, Menchola M. The efficacy of motivational interviewing: A meta-analysis of controlled clinical trials. *Journal of Consulting and Clinical Psychology*. 2003 Oct; 71:843–61.

Camarasa JG, Serra-Baldrich E, Lluch M, Malet A. Contact urticaria from sodium fluoride. *Contact Dermatitis*. 1993 May; 28:294.

Canadian Health Network (2003). Facts You Should Know About Smokeless (Spit) Tobacco. Retrieved August 21, 2005, from http://www.health.gov.sk.ca/rr_smokeless_tobacco.html

Chu CH, Lo ECM, Lin HC. Effectiveness of silver diamine fluoride and sodium fluoride varnish in arresting dentin caries in Chinese pre-school children. *Journal of Dental Research*. 2002 Nov; 81:767–70.

Cohen A, Weinstein P, Wurster C. Comparison of three confirmation systems with varying levels of patient responsibility in reducing broken appointments. *Journal of Dental Research*, 1978 Jan; 57(A):157.

Cousins MJ, Mazze RI. Methoxyfluorane nephrotoxicity: A study of dose-response in man. *Journal of the American Medical Association*. 1973 Sep; 225:1611–16.

Davies AR, Ware JE Jr. Measuring patient satisfaction with dental care. *Social Science and Medicine*. 1981 Dec; 15:751–60.

Derks A, Katsaros C, Frencken JE, van't Hoff MA, Kuijpers-Jagtman AM. Caries-inhibiting effect of preventive measures during orthodontic treatment with fixed appliances. A systematic review. *Caries Research*. 2004 Sept-Oct; 38:413–20.

Ekstrand J, Koch G, Petersson LG. Plasma fluoride concentration and urinary fluoride excretion in children following application of the fluoride containing varnish Duraphat. *Caries Research*. 1980; 14:185–9.

Featherstone JD, Adair SM, Anderson MH, Berkowitz RJ, Bird WF, Crall JJ, Den Besten PK, Donly KJ, Glassman P, Milgrom P, Roth

JR, Snow R, Stewart RE. Caries management by risk assessment: Consensus statement, April 2002. *Journal of the California Dental Association.* 2003 Mar; 31:257–69.

Geiger AM, Gorelick L, Gwinnett AJ, Benson BJ. Reducing white spot lesions in orthodontic populations with fluoride rinsing. *American Journal of Orthodontics and Dentofacial Orthopedics.* 1992 May; 101:403–7.

Golletz D, Milgrom P, Mancl L. Dental care satisfaction: the reliability and validity of the DSQ in a low-income population. *Journal of Dental Public Health.* 1995 Fall; 55:210–7.

Gorelick L, Geiger AM, Gwinnett AJ. Incidence of white spot formation after bonding and banding. *American Journal of Orthodontics,* 1982 Feb; 81:93–8.

Gotjamanos T. Safety issues related to the use of silver fluoride in paediatric dentistry. *Australian Dental Journal.* 1997 June; 42:166–8.

Hall, VR *et al.* Use of self-imposed contingencies to reduce the frequency of smoking behavior. Paper presented to the Association for Advancement of Behavioral Therapy, Washington D.C., 1971 Sept.

Heintze SD, Jost-Brinkmann PG, Loundos J. Effectiveness of three different types of electric toothbrushes compared with a manual technique in orthodontic patients. *American Journal of Orthodontics and Dentofacial Orthopedics.* 1996 Dec; 110:630–8.

Helfenstein U, Steiner M. Fluoride varnishes (Duraphat): A meta-analysis. *Community Dentistry and Oral Epidemiology.* 1994a Feb; 22:1–5.

Helfenstein U, Steiner, M. A note concerning the caries preventive effect of Duraphat. *Community Dentistry and Oral Epidemiology.*1994b Feb; 22.6–7.

Hensten-Pettersen A, Jacobsen N. Possible side effects related to dental hygienists' treatment. *Acta Odontologica Scandanavia.* 1994 Jun; 52:157–161.

Ho HP, Niederman R. Effectiveness of the Sonicare sonic toothbrush on reduction of plaque, gingivitis, probing pocket depth and subgingival bacteria in adolescent orthodontic patients. *Journal of Clinical Dentistry,* 1997 (1 Spec No); 8:15–19.

Isaksson M, Bruze M, Björkner B, Niklasson B. Contact allergy to Duraphat. *Scandanavian Journal of Dental Research,* 1993 Feb;

101:49-51.

Isotupa KP, Gunn S, Chen CY, Lopatin D, Makinen KK. Effect of polyol gums on dental plaque in orthodontic patients. *American Journal of Orthodontics and Dentofacial Orthopedics*. 1995 May; 107:497–504.

Iwata BA, Becksfort CM. Behavioral research in preventive dentistry: Educational and contingency management approaches to the problem of patient compliance. *Journal of Applied Behavior Analysis*. 1981 Summer; 14:111–20.

Koerber A, Crawford J, O'Connell K. The effects of teaching dental students brief motivational interviewing for smoking-cessation counseling: A pilot study. *Journal of Dental Education*. 2003 Apr; 67:439–47.

Lang NP, Cumming BR, Loe H. Toothbrushing frequency as it relates to plaque development and gingival health. *Journal of Periodontology*. 1973 July; 7:396–405.

Li YJ. Effect of a silver ammonia fluoride solution on the prevention and inhibition of caries. *Zhonghua Kou Qiang Ke Za Zhi*. 1984 June; 19:97–100.

Loe H, Theilade E, Jensen SB. Experimental gingivitis in man. Journal Periodontal Research. 1965 May-Jun; 36:177–87.

Loe H, von der Fehr FR, Schiott CR. Inhibition of experimental caries by plaque prevention. The effect of chlorhexidine mouthrinses. *Scandanavian Journal of Dental Research*. 1972; 80:1–9.

Ly KA, Milgrom P, Rothen M. Xylitol, sweeteners and dental caries. *Pediatric Dentistry*. 2006; 28: 154–63.

Machen DE. Legal aspects of orthodontic practice: Risk management concepts. The need for a structured dismissal plan. *American Journal of Orthodontics and Dentofacial Orthopedics*. 1990 Feb; 97:176–7.

Marcusson A, Norevall LI, Persson M. White spot reduction when using glass ionomer cement for bonding in orthodontics: a longitudinal and comparative study. *European Journal of Orthodontics*. 1997 June; 19(3):233–42.

Milgrom P, Rothen M, Spadafora A, Skaret E. A case report: Arresting dental caries. *Journal of Dental Hygiene*. 2001 Summer; 75:241–3.

Milgrom P, Weinstein P, Getz T. *Treating Fearful Dental Patients*, Second Edition. Seattle: Continuing Dental Education, University of Washington, 1995, 359 pp.

Moritani Y, Doi M, Yao K, Yoshihara M, Miyazaki K, Ito M, et al. Clinical evaluation of diamine silver fluoride (Saforide) in controlling caries of deciduous teeth. *Rinsho Shika*, 1970; 266:48–55.

Narrow WE. One-year prevalence of mental disorders, excluding substance use disorders, in the U.S.: NIMH ECA prospective data. Population estimates based on U.S. Census estimated residential population age 18 and over on July 1, 1998. Unpublished. Retrieved December 3, 2005, from http://www.nimh.nih.gov/publicat/numbers.cfm#1

National Cancer Institute. (2003). Smokeless Tobacco and Cancer: Questions and Answers. Retrieved August 21, 2005, from http://cis.nci.nih.gov/fact/10_15.htm

National Health Interview Survey (NHIS), 1999–2001. *Centers for Disease Control and Prevention*, National Center for Health Statistics, United States 2003 and 2004.

National Institute of Dental and Craniofacial Research, National Institutes of Health, U.S. Public Health Service, Department of Health and Human Services. The invisible barrier: literacy and its relationship with oral health. A report of a workgroup sponsored by the National Institute of Dental and Craniofacial Research, National Institutes of Health, U.S. Public Health Service, Department of Health and Human Services. *Journal of Public Health Dentistry* 2005, 65(3):174–82.

Neesham DC. Fluoride concentration in AgF and dental fluorosis. *Australian Dental Journal*, 1997 Aug; 42:268–9.

Nishino M, Yoshida S, Sobue S, Kato J. Effect of topically applied ammoniacal silver fluoride on dental caries in children. *Journal of Osaka University Dental School*. 1969 Sep; 9:149–55.

Nolan JD. Self-control procedures in the modification of smoking. Journal of Consulting and Clinical Psychology, 1968 Feb; 32:92–3.

Northwest/Alaska Center to Reduce Oral Health Disparities. EthnoDent: Bridging Sociocultural Boundaries in Children's Oral Health. Retrieved December 4, 2005 from http://depts.washington. edu/nacrohd/ethnodent/.

Nurenberger SI, Zimmerman J. Applied analyses of human behavior: An alternative to conventional motivational influences and unconscious determination in therapeutic programming. *Behavior*

Therapy, 1970; 1:59–69.

Ockene IS, Miller NH. *Cigarette smoking, cardiovascular disease, and stroke: a statement for healthcare professionals from the American Heart Association*. American Heart Association Task Force on Risk Reduction. Circulation. 1997 Nov 4; 96:3242–7.

Ogaard B. Prevalence of white spot lesions in 19-year-olds: a study on untreated and orthodontically treated persons 5 years after treatment. *American Journal of Orthodontics and Dentofacial Orthopedics*. 1989 Nov; 96:423–7.

Parker DR. A dental hygienists' role in tobacco cessation. *International Journal of Dental Hygiene*. 2003 May; 1(2):105–9.

Persson GR, Mancl LA, Martin J, Page RC. Assessing periodontal disease risk: A comparison of clinicians' assessment versus a computerized tool. *Journal of the American Dental Association*, 2003 May; 134:575–82.

Plotzitza B, Kneist S, Berger J, Hetzer G. Efficacy of chlorhexidine varnish applications in the prevention of early childhood caries. *European Journal of Paediatric Dentistry*. 2005 Sep; 6:149–54.

Ramsay DS. Patient compliance with oral hygiene regimens: A behavioural self-regulation analysis with implications for technology. *International Dental Journal*. 2000; 50:304–11.

Reibel J. Tobacco and oral diseases. Update on the evidence, with recommendations. *Medical Principles and Practice*. 2003; 12, Suppl.1:22–32.

Ricketts D. The eyes have it. How good is DIAGNOdent at detecting caries? *Evidence Based Dentistry*. 2005; 6:64–5.

Robinson PG, Deacon SA, Deery C, Heanue M, Walmsley AD, Worthington HV, Glenny AM, Shaw WC. Manual versus powered toothbrushing for oral health. *The Cochrane Database of Systemic Reviews* 2005, Issue 2. Art. No: CD002281.pub.2 DOI:10.1002/14651858.CD002281.pub2.

Sengun A, Sari Z, Ramoglu SI, Malkoc S, Duran L. Evaluation of the dental plaque pH recovery effect of a xylitol lozenge on patients with fixed orthodontic appliances. *The Angle Orthodontist*. 2004 Apr; 74:240–4.

Stalker CA, Russell BD, Teram E, Schachter CL. Providing dental care to survivors of childhood sexual abuse: Treatment considerations for the practitioner. *Journal of the American Dental Association*. 2005 Sep; 136:1277–81.

Stecksen-Blicks C, Holgerson PL, Olsson M, Bylund B, Sjostrom I, Skold-Larsson K, Kalfas S, Twetman S. Effect of xylitol on mutans streptococci and lactic acid formation in saliva and plaque from adolescents and young adults with fixed orthodontic appliances. *European Journal of Oral Sciences.* 2004 Jun; 112:244–8.

Tilashalski K, Rodu B, Cole P. A pilot study of smokeless tobacco in smoking cessation. *American Journal of Medicine,* 1998 May; 104:456–8.

Tilliss TS, Stach DJ, Cross-Poline GN, Annan SD, Astroth DB, Wolfe P. The Transtheoretical Model applied to an oral self-care behavioral change: Development and testing of instruments for stages of change and decisional balance. *Journal of Dental Hygiene.* 2003 Winter; 77:16–25.

Todd MA, Staley RN, Kanellis MJ, Donly K, Wefel JS. Effect of a fluoride varnish on demineralization adjacent to orthodontic brackets. *American Journal of Orthodontics and Dentofacial Orthopedics.* 1999 Aug; 116:159–67.

Twetman S, Petersson LG. Comparison of the efficacy of three different chlorhexidine preparations in decreasing the levels of mutans streptococci in saliva and interdental plaque. *Caries Research.* 1998; 32:113–8.

Walker EA, Milgrom P, Weinstein P, Getz T, Richardson R. Assessing abuse and neglect and dental fear in women. *Journal of the American Dental Association.* 1996 Apr; 127:485–90.

Weinstein, P. *Motivate your dental patients: A workbook.* University of Washington, Seattle, 2002.

Weinstein P, Fiset L. Long term assessment of a behavioral approach in plaque control using a multiple baseline design. Journal of Dental Research. 1983; 62:269.

Weinstein P, Harrison R, Benton T. Motivating parents to prevent caries in their young children. *Journal of the American Dental Association,* 2004 Jun; 135:731–38.

Weinstein P, Harrison R, Benton T, Motivating mothers to prevent caries: Confirming the beneficial effects of counseling, *Journal of the American Dental Association,* 2006 June 137.789–93

Whitford GM. *The metabolism and toxicity of fluoride.* 2nd Ed. Monographs in Oral Science, Vol. 16, Basel, Karger, 1996.

Wilson TG. How patient compliance to suggested oral hygiene and maintenance affect periodontal therapy. *Dental Clinics of North*

America. 1998 Apr; 42:389–403.

Winn DM. Tobacco use and oral disease. *Journal of Dental Education*. 2001 Apr; 65:306–12.

Yamaga R, Nishino N, Yoshida S, Yokomizo I. Diamine silver fluoride and its clinical application. *Journal of Osaka University Dental School*. 1972 Sep; 12:1–20.

Zickert I, Lindvall AM, Axelsson P. Effect on caries and gingivitis of a preventive program based on oral hygiene measures and fluoride application. *Community Dentistry and Oral Epidemiology*. 1982 Dec; 10:289–95.

Appendix

Caries Risk Management

CARIES RISK ASSESSMENT FORM FOR AGE 0 TO 5 YEARS

Patient Name:__________________ I.D. #______ Age ____ Date ____________

Initial/baseline exam date_______________ Recall/POE date ________________

Respond to each question in sections 1, 2, and 3 with a check mark in the yes or no column	Yes	No	Notes
1. Caries Risk Indicators - Parent Interview**			
(a) Mother or primary caregiver has had active dental decay in the past 12 months			
(b) Child has recent dental restorations (see 3b below)			
(c) Continual bottle use - contains fluids other than water			
(d) Child sleeps with a bottle, or nurses on demand			
(e) Frequent (greater than three times daily) between-meal snacks of sugars/cooked starch/sugared beverages			
(f) Saliva-reducing factors are present, including: 1. medications (e.g., some for asthma or hyperactivity) 2. medical (cancer treatment) or genetic factors			
(g) Child has developmental problems			
(h) Parent and/or caregiver has low SES (Socio-economic status) and/or low health literacy			
(i) No dental home/episodic dental care			
2. Protective Factors/Indicators – Parent Interview			
(a) Child lives in a fluoridated community or takes fluoride supplements by slowly dissolving or as chewable tablets			
(b) Teeth cleaned with fluoridated toothpaste (pea size) daily			
(c) Mother/caregiver have no caries activity			
(d) Mother/caregiver chews/sucks xylitol chewing gum/lozenges 2-4 X daily			
(e) Child has a dental home and regular dental care			
3. Caries Risk Indicators - Clinical Examination of Child**			
(a) Obvious white spots, decalcifications, or obvious decay present on the child's teeth			
(b) Restorations placed in the last 2 years			
(c) Plaque is obvious on the teeth and/or gums bleed easily			
(d) Dental or orthodontic appliances present, fixed or removable: e.g., braces, space maintainers, obturators			
(e) Visually inadequate saliva flow - dry mouth			

****If yes to any one of 1(a), 1(b), 3(a) or 3(b) or any two of 1(c)-1(i), or 3(c)-3(e), consider performing bacterial culture on mother or caregiver and child. Use this as a baseline to follow results of antibacterial intervention.**	Parent/Caregiver Date:	Child Date:
(a) Mutans streptococci (Indicate bacterial level: High, Medium, Low)		
(b) Lactobacillus species (Indicate bacterial level: High, Medium, Low)		

Child's overall caries risk status: (CIRCLE)	High	Moderate	Low

Recommendations given: yes______ no: ________ Date given:_______ or Date follow up:_______

Practitioner signature ________________________ Date: __________________

Instructions for Caries Risk Assessment Form – Children Ages 0 – 5 Years

1. **Answer the questions:** Respond to questions 1(a)–1(i), 2(a)–2(e) and 3(a)-3(e) with yes or no answers. You can make special notations such as the number of caries present, the severity of the lack of oral hygiene, the brand of fluorides used, the type of bottle contents used, the type of snacks eaten, or the names of medications/drugs that may be causing dry mouth.
2. **Determine the overall caries risk of the child:** Add up the yes answers to the high risk indicators from categories 1. and 3. Add up the number of yes answers for the protective factors/indicators, category 2. Make a judgment as to low, medium or high overall caries risk based on the balance between the pathological factors (caries risk indicators) and the protective factors. **Note:** Determining the caries risk for an individual child requires evaluating the number and severity of the risk indicators, not just the number. Certainly a child with caries presently or in the recent past is at high risk for future caries. A patient with low bacterial levels would need to have several other risk factors present to be considered at moderate risk. Some clinical judgment is needed while also considering the protective factors to determine the risk.
3. **Treatment Plan:** Treatment plan the case and decide what antibacterial therapy and fluoride treatments to use. High risk generally indicates that antibacterial therapy as well as additional fluoride therapy are both needed.
4. If the answer is yes to any one of 1(a), 1(b), 3(a) or 3(b) strongly consider using antibacterial therapy for mother/caregiver and the child.
5. Decide what restorative work is needed.
6. **Bacteria testing:** If the answer is yes to any one of 1(a), 1(b), 3(a) or 3(b), or any two of 1(c)-1(i), or 3(c)-3(e), consider performing bacterial cultures on mother or caregiver and child (see **notes in the form). See separate sheet for instructions how to perform these tests. Use these results as a baseline to follow the results of antibacterial intervention and whether to carry out antibacterial therapy for the mother/caregiver or child.
7. **Homecare recommendations:** Fill out the parent/care giver recommendation sheet based on your clinical observations and the responses to the questions and discuss strategies for caries control and management. Give one copy to the parent/caregiver and keep one in the patient's chart. Give the parent/caregiver the sheet that explains how caries happens (on the back of the home care recommendation sheet).
8. Place the completed caries risk assessment form in the patient's chart.
9. **Bacteria test results:** After the tests have incubated (72 hours, see separate instructions) inform the parent/care giver of the results of the bacteria tests. e.g. showing the parent the bacteria grown from their mouth (CRT test result) can be a good motivator so have the culture tube handy at the next visit (or schedule one for this purpose - the culture keeps satisfactorily for some weeks), or give/send them a picture, as a photograph or digital image. If the parent/care giver has high cariogenic bacterial counts then work with them and their own dentist to bring them to low caries risk and get their caries under

control to eliminate this source of infection and re-infection for the child.

10. **Follow up:** After the parent/care giver/child has been following your recommendations for 3-6 months, have them back to re-assess how well they are doing. Ask them if they are following your instructions – how often. If the bacterial levels were moderate or high initially, repeat the bacterial culture to see if bacterial levels have been reduced by antibacterial therapy. Make changes in your recommendations or reinforce protocol if results are not as good as desired or the patient is not compliant.

Bacterial testing:

Bacterial tests for cariogenic bacteria: There are two test kits currently available in the USA for "chair-side" testing for cariogenic bacterial challenge. One is the Caries Risk Test (CRT) marketed by Vivadent/Ivoclar (Amherst, NY). The other is the "Dentocult SM" and "Dentocult LB" test, marketed by Edge Dental (www.edgedental.com). Both are is sufficiently sensitive to provide a level of low, medium or high cariogenic bacterial challenge separately for mutans stereptococci (MS) and for lactobacilli species (LB). Each has selective media culture "sticks" that test MS and LB levels in saliva sampled from the patient. The CRT kit has a single "media stick" with selective media for MS on one side and LB on the other. The Dentocult slides come as two separate sticks. The results obtained from the test sticks from either supplier can also be used as a motivational tool for patient compliance with an antibacterial regimen. Other bacterial test kits will likely be available in the near future.

The following is the procedure for administering the currently available CRT test. Results are available after 72 hours.

The kit comes with two-sided selective media sticks that assess mutans streptococci on the blue side and lactobacilli on the green side. A starter kit , which includes plastic beakers, incubator and kits of 6 tests is available (Ivoclar catalog #NA 6556001). Manufacturers instructions are provided with each kit of 6 "media sticks". However, incubation for 72 hours rather than the recommended 48 hours, gives better results. The procedure can readily be done in a dental office or community clinic setting.

a) For mother/caregiver and for children old enough to spit (probably 4 or 5 years old), then a bacterial culture should be taken, as follows: The subject chews on the chewing gum (wax) provided in the kit for 3 minutes (accurately timed) and spits all mixed saliva into a measuring beaker. Measure the volume {in ml) and divide by 3 to give ml/minute stimulated saliva flow rate. Normal flow is greater than 1 ml/minute and low is less than 0.7 ml/minute.
b) Remove the selective media stick from the culture tube. Peel off the plastic sheet covering each side of the stick. Pour the collected saliva over the media on each side until it is entirely wet.
c) Place one of the sodium bicarbonate tablets (included with the kit) in the bottom of the tube.
d) Replace the media stick in the culture tube, screw the lid on and label the tube with the patient's name, number, and date.

e) Place the tube in the incubator at 37 ˚C for 72 hours. (Incubators suitable for a dental office are sold by the company).

f) Collect the tube after 72 hours and compare the densities of bacterial colonies with the pictures provided in the kit indicating relative bacterial levels, ranging from low to high. Colony densities in the middle of the range are medium. The dark blue agar is selective for mutans streptococci and the light green agar is selective for Lactobacilli. Record the level of bacterial challenge in the patient's chart, as low medium or high.

Bacteria testing for young children: For children not old enough to spit (aged 3 years or less) the bacterial levels of the parent/caregiver should be used as a rough estimate of the child's likely bacterial challenge. Children aged 0-3 years are difficult to culture reliably in the fashion described above. However a good approximate indication for the child can be obtained by using a cotton swab to sample the surfaces of all teeth and gums in the mouth, thoroughly dispersing the sample in about 1-2 ml of sterile saline in a test tube (Fisher Scientific), and dispersing it for 1 minute on a laboratory vortex (Fisher Scioentific, catalog 12-813-52). The suspension is then coated on the CRT stick as described above for saliva samples, and incubated for 72 hours. This will give a good estimate of the MS and LB challenge in the young child (Fujino *et al.*, 2004).

Parent/Caregiver Recommendations for Control of Dental Decay in Children 0-5 years

Daily Oral Hygiene/Fluoride Treatment *(These procedures reduce the bacteria in the mouth and provide a small amount of fluoride to guard against further tooth decay, as well as to repair early decayed areas.)*

___ brush child's teeth with a fluoride-containing toothpaste (small smear or pea-sized amount on a soft small infant sized toothbrush) twice daily (gently brushed by parent or caregiver)

___ selective daily flossing of areas with early caries (white patches)

___other: ______________________________

Diet (The aim is to reduce the number of between meal sweet snacks that contain carbohydrates, especially sugars. Substitution by snacks rich in protein, such as cheese will also help)

____ OK as is

____ limit bottle/nursing (to avoid prolonged contact of milk with teeth)

____ replace juice or sweet liquids in the bottle with water

____ limit snacking (particularly sweets)

____ replace high carbohydrate snacks with cheese and protein snacks

____ other ______________________________

Xylitol (Xylitol is a sweetener that the bacteria can not feed on. It limits the transfer of decay-causing bacteria from parent/caregiver to baby/toddler . Parents/caregivers with dental decay place their children at high risk. Parent/caregiver requires antibacterial treatment (see below). Using xylitol-containing chewing gum or mints/lozenges is a way that parents/caregivers of high risk children can use to reduce the transfer of decay-causing bacteria. This is most effective when used starting shortly after the child's birth.)

____ Parents of children 3 and under with high bacterial levels should use xylitol mints or xylitol gum 2–4 times daily

Antibacterial rinse (parents/caregivers)

____ Parents/caregivers of children 3 years and under with high bacterial levels should rinse with 10 ml of Chlorhexidine gluconate 0.12% (***Periogard, Peridox, Oral Rx*** by prescription only). Rinse at bedtime for 1 minute 1X/day for one week. Repeat each month for one week until infection is controlled. Continue for 6 months, or until bacterial levels remain controlled.

Practitioner signature ______________________ Date: ________________

Parent/careiver signature ______________________ Date: ______________

How Tooth Decay Happens

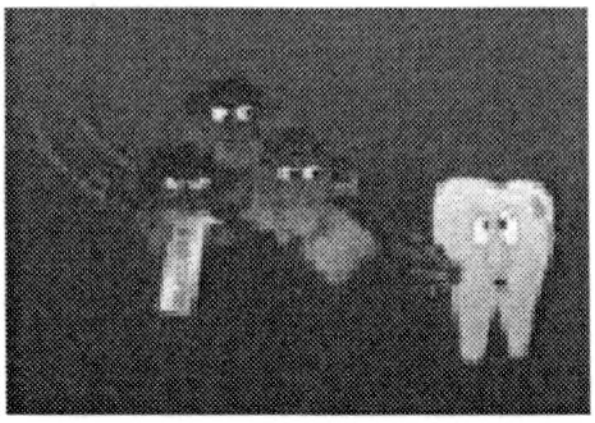

Tooth decay is caused by certain types of bacteria (bugs) that live in your mouth. When they stick to the film on your teeth called dental plaque, they can do damage. The bacteria feed on what you eat, especially sugars (including fruit sugars) and cooked starch (bread, potatoes, rice, pasta, etc.). Within about 5 minutes after you eat, or drink, the bacteria begin making acids as they digest your food. Those acids can break into the outer surface of the tooth and melt away some of the minerals. Your spit can balance the acid attacks if they don't happen very often. However if: 1) your mouth is dry, 2) you have a lot of these bacteria, or 3) you snack frequently; then acid causes loss of tooth minerals. This is the start of tooth decay and leads to cavities.

Methods of Controlling Tooth Decay

Diet: Reducing the number of sugary and starchy foods, snacks, or drinks can help reduce tooth decay. That does not mean you can never eat these types of foods. You should limit the times you eat these foods between main meals. A good rule is 3 meals per day and no more than 3 snacks per day.

Fluorides: Fluorides help to make teeth stronger and to protect against tooth decay, and to heal tooth decay if it has not gone too far. Fluorides are available from a variety of sources such as drinking water, toothpaste and rinses you can buy in the supermarket or drug store. They may also be prescribed by your dentist or applied in the dental office. Daily use of fluoride is very important to help protect against the acid attacks.

Plaque removal: Plaque is a yellowish film that sticks to the surface of teeth. Tooth brushing removes plaque and should be done every day. Bacteria live in plaque, so removing the plaque from your teeth on a daily basis helps to control tooth decay. Plaque is very sticky and may be hard to remove from between the teeth and in grooves on the biting surfaces of back teeth. If your child has an orthodontic retainer be sure to remove it before brushing your child's teeth. Brush all surfaces of the retainer also.

Spit: Spit (saliva) is important for healthy teeth. It balances acids, and provides other ingredients that protect the teeth. If you cannot brush after a meal or snack, you can chew sugar-free gum. This will stimulate the flow of saliva to help reduce the effect of acids. Sugar-free candy or mints can also be used, but some of these contain acids themselves. Acids in sugar-free candy will not cause tooth decay, but can slowly dissolve the tooth surface over time (a process called erosion). Some sugar-free gums are made to help fight tooth decay. Some gums contain baking soda that neutralizes the acids produced by the bacteria in plaque. **Gum that contains Xylitol as its first listed ingredient is the gum of choice**. This type of gum has been shown to protect against tooth decay and to reduce the decay causing bacteria.

Antibacterial mouth rinses: Rinses that your dentist can prescribe are able to reduce the numbers of bacteria that cause tooth decay and can be useful in patients at high risk for tooth decay. These rinses are only recommended for children who can rinse and spit.

Sealants: Sealants are plastic coatings brushed onto the biting surfaces of back teeth to protect the deep grooves from decay. In some people the grooves on the surfaces of the teeth are too narrow and deep to clean with a toothbrush. They may decay even if you brush them regularly. Sealants are an excellent preventive measure used for children and young adults at risk for this type of decay.

CARIES RISK ASSESSMENT FORM CHILDREN - AGED 6 YEARS AND OVER/ADULTS

Patient Name:____________________ I.D. #______ Age ____ Date ____________

Initial/baseline exam date_________________ Recall/POE date _________________

			Notes
Respond to <u>each</u> questions in sections 1, 2 and 3 with a check mark in the yes or no column	yes	no	
1. High Risk Factors**			
(a) Visible cavitation (carious) or caries into dentin by radiograph			
(b) Caries restored in last 3 years			
(c) readily visible heavy plaque on teeth			
(d) Frequent (greater than 3 times daily) between meal snacks of sugars/cooked starch			
(e) **Saliva reducing factors:**			
1. hyposalivatory medications			
2. radiation to head and neck			
3. systemic reasons, e.g. Sjogren's			
(f*) Visually inadequate saliva flow. **(If yes, measure)** less than 0.7 ml/min by test = low salivary flow or dry mouth			Amount: _______ml/min
(g) appliances present, fixed or removable: e.g. orthodontic brackets/bands/ retainer or removable partial denture(s)			
2. Moderate Risk Factors			
(a) exposed roots			
(b) deep pits & fissures/developmental defects			
(c) interproximal enamel lesions/radiolucencies			
(d) other white spot lesions or occlusal discoloration			
(e) Uses recreational drugs			
3. Protective Factors			
(a) lives/works/school in fluoridated community			
(b) uses fluoride toothpaste daily			type ______________
(c) uses fluoride mouthwash/rinse/gel daily			type ______________
(d*) Salivary flow visually adequate or >1 ml/min by test			Amount: _______ml/min
(e) Uses xylitol gum or mints 4 x day			Type ____and % xylitol_____
(f) Uses chlorhexidine rinse			Brand________Frequency.

****If yes to 1(a) or any two of 1(b)–(g), perform bacterial culture***	**High Count** Date:_____	**Moderate Count** Date:______	**Low Count** Date:_____	
(a) mutans streptococci				(Place a check in the box below count)
(b) Lactobacillus				(Place a check in the box below count)
Caries Risk-overall*(see over)	**High**	**Moderate**	**Low**	**<u>Circle High, Moderate or Low</u>**
Recommendations given: Yes _____ No ______			Date given:_____or Date follow up:____	

<u>*Indicates that test descriptions for these procedures are on the following page</u>

Instructions for Caries Risk Assessment Form – Children Ages 6 Years and over/Adults

1. Respond to questions 1,2,3 with yes or no answers. You can make special notations such as the number of caries present, the severity of the lack of oral hygiene, the brand of fluorides used, the type of snacks eaten, or the names of medications/drugs that are causing dry mouth.
2. If the answer is yes to question 1(a) or any two of questions 1(b)-1(g), then a bacterial culture should be taken using the **CRT bacteria test*** (Vivadent) – see below. Make an overall judgment as to whether the patient is at high, medium or low risk dependent on the balance between the pathological factors (sections 1 and 2) and the protective factors (section 3). **Note!** Determining the caries risk for an individual requires evaluating the number and severity of the risk factors. Certainly an individual with caries presently or in the recent past is at high risk for future caries. A patient with low bacterial levels would need to have several other risk factors present to be considered at moderate risk. Some clinical judgment is needed while also considering the protective factors to determining the risk. **Note!** Children with developmental problems or low socio-economic status (SES) are automatically at high risk. Have the faculty check your work, and place the completed form in the patient chart.
3. Provide the patient with recommendations based on your clinical observations and the responses to the questions and discuss strategies for caries control and management. Give the patient the sheet that explains how caries happens and the sheet with your recommendations. Copy the recommendations for the patient chart.
4. Inform the patient of the results of any test results. e.g., showing the patient the bacteria grown from their mouth (CRT test result*) can be a good motivator so have the culture tube handy at the next visit (or schedule one for this purpose - the culture keeps satisfactorily for some weeks), or give/send them a picture.
5. After the patient has been following your recommendations for 3-6 months, have the patient back to re-assess how well they are doing. Ask them if they are following your instructions – how often. If the bacterial levels were moderate or high initially, repeat the bacterial culture to see if bacterial levels have been reduced. Make changes in your recommendations or reinforce protocol if results are not as good as desired or the patient is not compliant.

*Test procedures – Saliva Flow Rate and Caries Bacteria Testing

*1. *Saliva Flow Rate:* Have the patient chew a paraffin pellet (included with the CRT test – see below) for 3-5 minutes (timed) and spit all saliva generated into a cup. At the end of the 3-5 minutes measure the amount of saliva (in milliliters = ml) and divide that amount by time to determine the ml/minute of stimulated salivary flow. A flow rate of 1ml/min and above is considered normal. A level of 0.7 ml/min is low and anything at 0.5 ml/min or less is dry, indicating a high risk situation. Investigation of the reason for the low flow rate is an important step in the patient treatment.

*2. ***Bacterial testing:*** **CRT bacteria test:** In the USA the currently available "chair-side" test for cariogenic bacterial challenge is the Caries Risk Test (CRT) marketed by Vivadent (Amherst, NY). It is sufficiently sensitive to provide a level of low, medium or high cariogenic bacterial challenge. It can also be used as a motivational tool for patient compliance with an antibacterial regimen. Other bacterial test kits will likely be available in the near future. The following is the procedure for administering the currently available CRT test. Results are available after 48 hours.

The kit comes with two-sided selective media sticks that assess mutans streptococci on the blue side and lactobacilli on the green side.

a) Remove the selective media stick from the culture tube. Peel off the plastic cover sheet from each side of the stick.
b) Pour the collected saliva over the media on each side until it is entirely wet.
c) Place one of the sodium bicarbonate tablets (included with the kit) in the bottom of the tube.
d) Replace the media stick in the culture tube, screw the lid on and label the tube with the patient's name, registration number, and date. Place the tube in the incubator at 37°C for 72 hours. Incubators suitable for a dental office are also sold by the company.
e) Collect the tube after 72 hours and compare the densities of bacterial colonies with the pictures provided in the kit indicating relative bacterial levels. The dark blue agar is selective for mutans streptococci and the light green agar is selective for Lactobacilli. Record the level of bacterial challenge in the patient's chart, as low medium or high.

Patient Recommendations for Control of Dental Decay (Ages 6 and over/adult)

Daily Oral Hygiene *(Aimed at reducing the overall bacteria in the mouth, especially at sites likely to decay. Choose the recommendations based on the danger sites and the condition of the mouth.)*

___ brush twice daily (with fluoride toothpaste, all patients) ____ floss daily
____ interproximal brush ____ Stimudents ____ toothpick ____ Superfloss
other: ____

Diet (The most important thing is to reduce the number of between meal sweet snacks that contain carbohydrates, especially sugars. Substitution by snacks rich in protein, such as cheese will also help)

____ OK as is ____ limit snacking ___ limit sodas ___ other ____________________.

Fluorides (All patients should use a fluoride toothpaste twice daily. Additional fluoride products should be added, depending on whether the risk level is medium or high. These fluoride products must be used daily to be effective)

____ fluoride-containing toothpaste 2X/day (all patients regardless of caries risk status)

____ fluoride rinse (0.05 % NaF, ***ACT*** or ***Fluorigard***) 1X or 2X/day (use in addition to toothpaste. Patients at medium risk should rinse in the morning or last thing at night. For high risk patients use twice a day, once in the morning and once last thing at night. Continue long term with older patients or those who need or want extra protection)

____ ***Prevident*** or *Control Rx* "brush-on" nightly, **OR** ____ gel (***Prevident***) in custom tray 10 min./night (For high risk patients, especially those with low saliva flow, or root caries, or active cavities. Continue until the risk status is lowered, then revert to fluoride as above)

____ fluoride lozenges (***Lozi-Flur*** or ***Fluor-a-day***) 1X/day (use for high risk patients with low saliva flow, such as radiation xerostomia. By dissolving in the mouth these lozenges provide a concentrated fluoride reservoir to protect against mineral loss and to enhance repair by remineralization. Dissolve slowly in mouth by holding the lozenge in a convenient place)

Sugar-free gum/mints (recommend for high risk patients, especially those with low saliva flow, and/or those who need to reduce in between meal snacking. The gums or mints that contain xylitol also have an antibacterial effect against the decay-causing bacteria Preferably use a xylitol-containing gum.)

____ Chew after meals when you can't brush (xylitol preferred).

____ Use Xylitol mints 3 – 4 times daily.

Antibacterial rinse

____ Chlorhexidine gluconate, 0.12% (***Periogard, Peridex, Oral Rx,*** available on prescription). Rinse with 10 ml at bedtime for 1 minute, 1X/day for one week. Repeat every month until infection is reduced to safe levels. Use fluoride rinse or high concentration F dentifrice (5000 ppm F) (see above) every day during the weeks in between.

For dry mouth

____ baking soda tooth paste with fluoride ____ baking soda gum - ***Dental Care Gum*** (Arm & Hammer. It contains baking soda and xylitol) or similar product. —Chew frequently throughout the day.

____ rinse frequently with baking soda suspension during the day (fill sports water bottle with water and add 2 teaspoons of baking soda for each 8 oz. of water.)

Practitioner signature ______________________ Date: ____________________

Patient signature ____________________________ Date ____________________

How Tooth Decay Happens

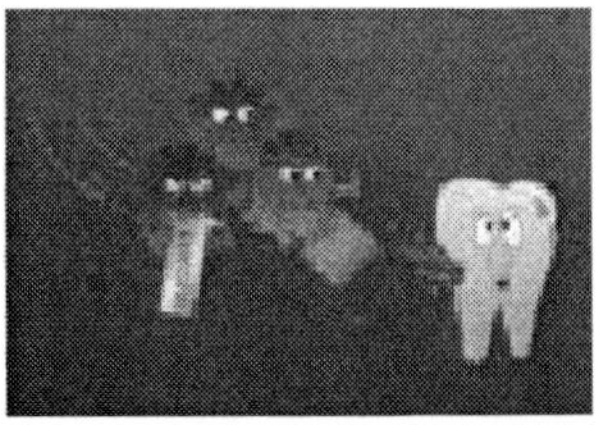

Tooth decay is caused by certain types of bacteria (mutans streptococci and Lactobacilli) that live in your mouth. When they attach themselves to the teeth and multiply in dental plaque, they can do damage. The bacteria feed on what you eat, especially sugars (including fruit sugars) and cooked starch (bread, potatoes, rice, pasta, etc.). Within about 5 minutes after you eat, or drink, the bacteria begin producing acids as a by-product of their digesting your food. Those acids can penetrate into the hard substance of the tooth and dissolve some of the minerals (calcium and phosphate). If the acid attacks are infrequent and of short duration, your saliva can help to repair the damage by neutralizing the acids and supplying minerals and fluoride that can replace those lost from the tooth. However if: 1) your mouth is dry, 2) you have many of these bacteria, or 3) you snack frequently; then the tooth mineral lost by attacks of acids is too great, and cannot be repaired. This is the start of tooth decay and leads to cavities.

Methods of Controlling Tooth Decay

Diet: Reducing the number of sugary and starchy foods, snacks, drinks or candies can help reduce the development of tooth decay. That does not mean you can never eat these types of foods, but you should limit their consumption particularly when eaten between main meals. A good rule is 3 meals per day and no more than 3 snacks per day.

Fluorides: Fluorides help to make the tooth more resistant to being dissolved by the bacterial acids. Fluorides are available from a variety of sources such as drinking water, toothpaste, over-the-counter rinses, and products prescribed by your dentist such as brush-on gels used at home or gels and foams applied in the dental office. Daily use is very important to help protect against the acid attacks.

Plaque removal: Removing the plaque from your teeth on a daily basis is helpful in controlling tooth decay. Plaque can be difficult to remove from some parts of your mouth especially between the teeth and in grooves on the biting surfaces of back teeth. If you have an appliance such as an orthodontic retainer or partial denture remove it before brushing your teeth. Brush all surfaces of the appliance also.

Saliva: Saliva is critical for controlling tooth decay. It neutralizes acids, and provides minerals and proteins that protect the teeth. If you cannot brush after a meal or snack, you can chew some sugar-free gum. This will stimulate the flow of saliva to help neutralize acids and bring lost minerals back to the teeth. Sugar-free candy or mints could also be used, but some of these contain acids themselves. These acids will not cause tooth decay, but they can slowly dissolve the enamel surface directly over time (a process called erosion). Some sugar-free gums are designed to help fight tooth decay and are particularly useful if you have a dry mouth (many medications can cause a dry mouth). Some gums contain baking soda that neutralizes the acids produced by the bacteria in plaque.

Gum that contains Xylitol as its first listed ingredient is the gum of choice. If you have a dry mouth, you could also fill a drinking bottle with water and add a couple tea spoons of baking soda for each 8 ounces of water and swish with it frequently throughout the day. Toothpastes containing baking soda are also available by several companies.

Antibacterial mouth rinses: Rinses that your dentist can prescribe are able to reduce the numbers of bacteria that cause tooth decay and can be useful in patients at high risk for tooth decay.

Sealants: Sealants are plastic coatings bonded to the biting surfaces of back teeth to protect the deep grooves from decay. In some people the grooves on the surfaces of the teeth are too narrow and deep to clean with a toothbrush, so they may decay in spite of your best efforts. Sealants are an excellent preventive measure used for children and young adults at risk for this type of decay.

Index

Exam Questions

Exam Questions for Chapter 1:

Why Most Plaque Programs Do Not Work

1. Which of the following is NOT true about the plaque-control programs introduced by dental professionals in the 1960's and early 1970's?
   A.. The programs resulted in long-term changes in patients' hygiene
   B. The programs resulted in rapid initial improvement in patients' hygiene
   C. Patients' hygiene tended to return to baseline levels after an initial improvement
   D. Changes in hygiene were not maintained without professional supervision
2. According to research studies, most patients who begin a preventative oral health program drop out of such programs within:
   A. Two weeks (14 days)
   B. Two months (60 days)
   C. Three months (90 days)
   D. Six months (180 days)
3. According to the authors, what is likely the best way to approach a patient about beginning a plaque-control program at home?
   A. "I can see that you haven't been taking as good care of your mouth as you could be."
   B. "If I could wave a magic wand and instantly change how your teeth look, how would you like them to look?"

   C. "How long has it been since you've had your teeth cleaned again?"
   D. "Let me show you how you should be brushing your teeth."
4. What is the most important aspect of the "message" that dental providers relate to patients?
   A. It is personalized and relevant to the patients' individual concerns
   B. It is technical and includes several scientific details
   C. It is presented in a concise manner that keeps the appointment short
   D. It involves providing several oral health tools and written materials
5. You have been seeing a 45-year-old patient for 3 years, and have spoken with him several times about the importance of flossing. At his most recent appointment, he admits to you that he has not been flossing regularly. The most likely reason for this lack of compliance is:
   A. He doesn't care enough about his oral health to floss
   B. You haven't given him enough floss to bring home and use
   C. You haven't given him enough reasons to floss
   D. He is unsure how to establish and maintain a long-term flossing behavior

Exam Questions for Chapter 2:

Communicating With Your Patients

1. Which of the following is a possible source of oral health information for patients?
   A. Family and friends
   B. Media sources (newspapers, television, etc.)
   C. Internet
   D. All of the above

2. A 32-year-old female patient tells you that she doesn't brush her teeth as often as she should because, in her words, "All of my teeth are going to fall out anyway, so why bother taking good care of them?" The best approach for this patient is:
   A. Dismiss her from your practice; if she insists on not taking care of her teeth, there's nothing you can do for her
   B. Give her additional instruction on how to brush properly
   C. Offer to discuss with her ways in which she may be able to keep her teeth
   D. Provide her with information about dentures and dental implants
3. Which of the following is NOT a good example of a "patient friendly" word or phrase for <u>adults</u>?
   A. discomfort
   B. having a tooth pulled
   C. cavity
   D. root canal
4. Your 65-year-old male patient appears upset after a procedure. Before he leaves your office, you ask him, "How was your filling today?" He responds, "it really start to hurt at the end, but I knew we were almost done, so I didn't say anything." You then discuss with him the use of hand signals to stop the procedure if he is in pain, and reassure him that he can stop any procedure at any time. Discussing earlier problems with patients so that they may plan ways to cope with treatment in the future is known as:
   A. Retrospective control
   B. Cognitive control
   C. Behavioral control
   D. Procedural control
5. A patient's past dental experiences:
   A. Should only be discussed if they were mostly positive; talking about bad experiences will only increase the patient's anxiety

B. Aren't important to current treatment; what's past is past
C. Should be acknowledged and used to tailor future treatment
D. Are only relevant if they keep you from completing treatment

Exam Questions for Chapter 3:

Therapeutic Alternatives

1. Topical fluoride varnish:
    A. Is widely used in the United States, but not in other countries
    B. Can arrest and remineralize damaged tooth structure
    C. Should not be used on "white spot" lesions
    D. Is only effective if carious lesions have developed into the dentin
2. Fluoride and chlorhexidine have different but compatible mechanisms of action. While fluoride ________________, chlorhexidine ________________.
    A. remineralizes teeth; is an antimicrobial
    B. whitens teeth; replaces flossing
    C. is an antimicrobial; remineralizes teeth
    D. replaces flossing; whitens teeth
3. Xylitol has been shown to be beneficial, particularly for patients with orthodontic or prosthetic appliances. The most effective dose has been shown to be _____ per day divided over at least ___ doses.
    A. 10 milligrams; 5
    B. 2 grams; 4
    C. 6 grams; 3
    D. 0.5 milligrams; 2
4. You diagnose a patient with periodontitis, and recommend gingival curettage and scaling and root planing at least 3 times within the next 12 months. The patient explains that she does not have the financial means to follow this treatment plan. What should you recommend?
    A. Consultation for full dentures
    B. Brushing and flossing at least 5 times per day

C. Periodontal treatment as recommended, but on a more limited scope
D. Periodontal treatment as recommended, but from a dental clinic that charges less than you do

5. You recommend chlorhexidine rinse for an adolescent female patient. She tries a taste in your office, then spits it back into the sink, saying, "That stuff is gross! I don't want to use that!" What is the best approach for this patient?
   A. Suggest an oral rinse that may not work as well, but tastes better
   B. Send the patient home with the chlorhexidine – she'll use it if her parents "bug" her enough
   C. Do not send the patient home with the chlorhexidine – she'll ask for it once she sees how bad her mouth looks without it.
   D. Arrange for the patient to come in for a cleaning more often until a consistent home program is established

Exam Questions for Chapter 4:

Motivating Patients

1. In addition to oral health care, Motivational Interviewing has been used successfully for all EXCEPT the following:
   A. Smoking
   B. Medication compliance
   C. Exercise
   D. It has been used successfully with all of the above

2. You speak with a patient about beginning a home program of daily flossing. He says, "I know I should floss more often, but my gums bleed so much when I do, and it takes so much time." After three months, he returns to your office and reports that he has been flossing twice a day for the last 3 weeks. According to the Transtheoretical Model of Change, this patient began in the _________ stage and is now in the ________ stage.
   A. precontemplative; maintenance
   B. contemplative; action

C. preparation; maintenance
D. precontemplative; action

3. Which of the following is TRUE about the Stages of Change?
    A. Individuals move in a "direct line" through the stages
    B. Individuals can move back and forth through the stages, depending on their readiness to change
    C. Individuals who do not move from one stage to another are in denial of their problems and must see a professional therapist to address their problems
    D. Individuals need to meet with a psychologist who is specifically trained in Motivational Interviewing in order to realize what Stage of Change they are in
4. Resistance:
    A. increases when dental providers offer unsolicited advice
    B. decreases when the advice benefits the patient
    C. decreases when the dental provider stresses that he/she is the "expert"
    D. increases when the provider gives the patient the power to decide for him/herself
5. Your patient says that although she wants to have her front teeth fixed, she feels guilty spending money on her teeth when she could use it to buy more things for her children. You respond, "It sounds like you're saying that while you want to improve the way your teeth look, you're not sure you want to spend this money on yourself. Did I get that right?" This is an example of:
    A. Restating
    B. Amplified reflection
    C. Double-sided reflection
    D. Reframing

Exam Questions for Chapter 5:

Teaching Skills

1. Research has shown that which tooth surface is LEAST likely to be cleaned while toothbrushing?
   A. Buccal
   B. Occlusal
   C. Lingual
   D. Labial

2. What seems to be the best way to structure oral health skill-teaching sessions?
   A. Four or five short sessions, with 5-10 minutes at each appointment for instruction
   B. One long session of instruction, working at it until the patient is proficient
   C. Two longer sessions of instruction, divided by a professional cleaning
   D. Twenty to thirty minutes of instruction every 6 months

3. When instructing patients on toothbrushing:
   A. The quantity of time spent brushing should be emphasized
   B. The quality of brushing should be emphasized
   C. Disclosing tablets are rarely helpful
   D. It is critical that patients are told to brush after every meal

4. The role of feedback in teaching new skills:
   A. Is only to provide information about what the patient is doing right
   B. Is to help transfer new skills from the office to the patient's home
   C. Is diminished when used in conjunction with written logs
   D. Is to make patients feel embarrassed about the "old way" of doing things

5. When teaching patients about interproximal cleaning:
   A. Patients should always be told to stop if bleeding occurs
   B. Floss is the "safest" form as it never causes damage to the gingiva

C. Patients should be reassured that bleeding will stop with continued interproximal cleaning
D. Focusing only on one spot at first will discourage patients from moving on to other areas of the mouth

Exam Questions for Chapter 6:

Planning to Collect Baseline Data

1. When collecting baseline data, all of the following may occur EXCEPT:
   A. The frequency of an unwanted behavior may decrease simply due to the fact that its frequency is being recorded
   B. The frequency of a desired behavior may decrease simply due to the fact that its frequency is being recorded
   C. A decision may be made not to begin a behavior change program after all
   D. Both the patient and dental provider may obtain a realistic idea of how often a behavior occurs

2. Which of the following is an important when beginning to collect baseline data?
   A. Identifying a behavior that can be observed and measured
   B. Pinpointing a behavior to monitor and record
   C. Determine in what situations the behavior is likely to occur
   D. All of the above

3. When is baserate counting NOT likely to be helpful?
   A. When the patient requires structure
   B. When the frequency of (how often) the behavior is important
   C. When the effectiveness of (how well) the behavior is important
   D. When the quantity of (how many times) the behavior is important

4. A 16-year-old female patient wishes to stop biting her fingernails. You speak with her about collecting baseline data, and she notes that she is much more likely to bite her fingernails while she is in Study Hall at school. You both decide that for a period of 2 weeks,

she will count the number of times she bites her nails during her daily Study Hall periods. This is an example of:

A. Counting the permanent products of behavior
B. Time sampling
C. Event recording
D. Interval recording

5. A baserate contract between a dental provider and patient:
   A. Should be changed as the needs and readiness of the patient change
   B. Should be developed by the provider and presented to the patient
   C. Is a legally binding contract
   D. Must be signed by the provider, patient, and independent witness

Exam Questions for Chapter 7:

Specific Goals and Objectives

1. In order to most effectively progress to the stage of specifying goals and objectives, the patient should be in the ________ or ______ Stage of Change.
   A. preparation; action
   B. precontemplative; maintenance
   C. contemplative; action
   D. maintenance; preparation

2. Which of the following is a good example of an intermediate goal?
   A. "I'm going to stop eating so much junk food."
   B. "I'm going to take better care of my teeth."
   C. "I'm going to walk around my neighborhood for 30 minutes, three times a week."
   D. "I've just got to stop smoking, or my husband/wife will kill me."

3. Which of the following is NOT true about choosing appropriate goals?
    A. You can never be too optimistic about a patient's ability to reach a goal
    B. Deciding on goals should be a team effort between the patient and provider
    C. Aiming "too high" will lead to patients feeling frustrated and giving up
    D. Aiming "too low" will lead to patients feeling bored and giving up
4. Your 17-year-old male patient acknowledges that he would like to wear his orthodontic retainer more often. Specifically, he would like to wear it for 3 hours a day after school; he currently wears it for about 1 hour every other day. What would be the best way to begin to shape the desired behavior?
    A. Set a goal for 3 hours every day and encourage the patient to meet this goal
    B. Set a goal for 30 minutes on the days he is currently not wearing the retainer
    C. Tell the patient to wear the retainer when he feels like it; he will wear it more often if it is his choice to do so
    D. Provide the patient with information about the consequences of not wearing his retainer
5. When should you tell a patient to move on to the next step of the behavior change?
    A. When a certain period of time has gone by
    B. When the patient gets frustrated at the earlier step
    C. When it seems like the patient "should" be ready to move on
    D. When the patient feels confident in his/her ability to maintain the behavior frequency at the earlier step

Exam Questions for Chapter 8:

Planning an Intervention

1. According to the authors, what is the most important factor influencing the strength of a particular behavior?
   A. A person's experiences leading up to when the behavior occurs
   B. The consequences of the behavior that occur over a long period of time after the behavior occurs
   C. The consequences of the behavior that occur immediately after the behavior occurs
   D. The antecedents that occur immediately before the behavior
2. Which of the following is NOT true about consequences of behavior?
   A. A particular consequence will increase or decrease behavior the same way for every person
   B. Consequences affect the likelihood that a behavior will happen because the individual finds the consequences that follow the behavior either desirable or undesirable
   C. We cannot always predict what effect a particular consequence will have
   D. A good time to identify consequences is when you or your patient are taking baseline counts of a behavior
3. Which of the following is a good example of an *antecedent* of a behavior?
   A. A patient complains to you that, "No matter how hard I brush, I still get cavities!"
   B. A patient sets out a container of floss next to his toothbrush and toothpaste to remind himself to floss
   C. A patient eats a large piece of cheesecake after dinner, and two days later, sees the numbers on her bathroom scale "inch up"
   D. A patient cuts down on the number of cigarettes he smokes in a day after his wife complains about the smell

4. According to the Premack Principle, which of the following is most likely to increase the frequency of a desired behavior?
   A. Pointing out all of the areas of a patient's mouth that are bleeding if he does not floss
   B. Requiring that a patient put $1 in a "flossing jar" for every day he does not floss
   C. Rewarding a patient for flossing by praising his improved oral health
   D. Requiring a patient to floss before he goes to play his daily basketball game.
5. It is obvious to you, through your examination, that your 35-year-old female patient has been flossing regularly. Before sending her home with additional floss and other oral care products, you mention to her that you're very pleased with her progress. This is an example of:
   A. Material reinforcement
   B. Actitvity reinforcement
   C. Material and social reinforcement
   D. Activity and material reinforcement

Exam Questions for Chapter 9:

Monitoring and Modifying the Plan

1. Which is the BEST example of what to say to a patient who has not followed through with his/her behavior change plan?
   A. "Let me go over again what you had planned to do."
   B. "Well, what went wrong?"
   C. "Could we talk a bit about what got in your way?"
   D. "Why don't we try this again in six months?"
2. You have been treating a child who frequently refuses to cooperate with treatment. He cries, refuses to open his mouth, and says he wants his mother in the operatory. You have tried reinforcing good behavior, but the child still misbehaves. According to the authors in this chapter, which of the following is the best approach for you to take?

A. Tell the child that his mother can stay in the operatory with him as long as he keeps his mouth open
B. Tell the child that if he does not keep his mouth open, his mother will be very upset with him
C. Try to distract the child with toys and games
D. Disregard the child's protests and proceed with treatment as planned

3. Which of the following is FALSE regarding problems in behavior change?
A. They are extremely common
B. They often occur early in the behavior change process
C. They are nearly always due to a lack of motivation
D. They can often be solved through good communication

4. Your 46-year-old female patient has been working on a home-care program that includes daily use of chlorhexidine. She reports to you that although she had been using the rinse daily for 4 weeks, she stopped using it a week ago because of staining and disagreeable taste. While she acknowledges that she saw some benefit to using the rinse, she is now not certain she wants to continue. With regard to the Stages of Change Model, it seems as though this patient was previously in the ______ stage, and is currently in the ______ stage.
A. maintenance; precontemplative
B. action; contemplative
C. contemplative; precontemplative
D. preparation; maintenance

5. Which of the following would be an acceptable response to a patient not keeping up with a behavior change program?
A. Reexamining the rewards used by the patient
B. Changing the frequency of rewards
C. Using the Premack Principle to increase the likelihood that the behavior will occur
D. All of the above

Exam Questions for Chapter 10:

Maintaining Change

1. A person must maintain a behavior change for ______ in order to move from the "action" to "maintenance" phase.
    A. Six weeks
    B. Three months
    C. Six months
    D. One year
2. Which of the following is TRUE about eliminating the reward and support systems in the maintenance phase?
    A. These systems should be stopped abruptly
    B. These systems should be gradually limited then stopped
    C. These systems should be maintained indefinitely
    D. These systems are not important in the behavior change process
3. The primary difference between a "lapse" and "relapse" is:
    A. A "relapse" is a decision to stop the behavior change, while a "lapse" is a brief return to the original behavior
    B. A "lapse" is a decision to stop the behavior change, while a "relapse" is a brief return to the original behavior
    C. A "relapse" is seen as normal and expected
    D. A "lapse" should be discouraged by all means necessary
4. A "booster session" during the maintenance phase:
    A. Should occur at the normal 6-month recall appointment
    B. Is only necessary if the patient shows signs of "relapsing" into the old behavior
    C. Should occur within 30 to 60 days of the initial treatment
    D. Should occur the first time a patient has a "lapse"
5. Which of the following is an acceptable form of maintaining a recall schedule with patients?
    A. Phone calls
    B. Postcards
    C. Email
    D. All of the above

Exam Questions for Chapter 11:

Tobacco Use – Helping Patients Quit

1. Which of the following is NOT true about smokeless tobacco?
   A. It is a safe alternative to smoking cigarettes or cigars
   B. Nicotine in smokeless tobacco enters the bloodstream more slowly than with cigarettes or cigars
   C. Smokeless tobacco contains abrasives and sugars that can damage teeth
   D. Use of smokeless tobacco has been linked to heart disease, oral and throat cancers, stomach ulcers and cancer

2. All of the following are forms of smokeless tobacco EXCEPT:
   A. Chew
   B. Plug
   C. Snuff
   D. Shred

3. You discuss quitting smoking with a 42-year-old male patient. He says that while he hates the taste of cigarettes as well as spending money on them, the only time he gets to talk to his friends at work is during their "smoke breaks." This is an example of _________, one of the reasons why people don't quit smoking.
   A. Nicotine addiction
   B. Social factors
   C. Environmental cues
   D. Behavioral aspects

4. Which of the following should you NOT encourage a patient to do if she is trying to quit smoking?
   A. Do other things with her hands when she would typically smoke
   B. Avoid or cut down on alcohol use
   C. Spend time with her friends who smoke so she will get used to being around smokers without smoking herself
   D. Do other things with his hands when he would typically smoke

5. Often, combining smoking cessation methods is helpful in allowing patients to quit. For example, _____ is a commonly used antidepressant medication that can help reduce withdrawal symptoms. Nicotine gum and lozenges are ____, while patients are advised to _____ while wearing a nicotine patch.
   A. Prozac; chewed for at least 10 minutes; avoid going swimming
   B. Buproprion; placed between the cheek and gums; avoid using tobacco products
   C. Buproprion; chewed for at least 10 minutes; avoid using tobacco products
   D. Prozac; placed between cheek and gums; avoid going swimming

Exam Questions for Chapter 12:

Oral Self-Care and Children

1. Which of the following is TRUE about children who experience a traumatic dental procedure?
   A. They eventually "grow out of" their fear as they get older
   B. They often become avoidant of dental care, requiring more invasive and extensive restorative care
   C. The initial trauma is usually caused by their poor cooperation during treatment
   D. They almost never develop dental fear as adults
2. Researchers have found that when anxious mothers attempt to _______ their children's anxieties, they paradoxically ______ anxiety.
   A. talk about; decrease
   B. increase; decrease
   C. manage; limit
   D. decrease; increase
3. Regarding allowing parents in the operatory, the authors state that the mother or father should be allowed to remain in the operatory

A. if the parent is not overtly anxious
B. if the parent helps the provider complete treatment
C. if the child repeatedly asks for his parent
D. If treatment cannot be accomplished any other way

4. Which of the following is NOT true about treating adolescents?
   A. They have a particularly strong desire to establish and maintain independence of action
   B. Because they are no longer children, they should always be treated just like adults
   C. They frequently do not perceive the worth of the preventive measures we expect them to perform
   D. They are often sensitive to criticism, and giving them feedback often results in conflict or avoidance

5. What is the primary difference between treating adolescents compared with treating children?
   A. Adolescents should be asked for input about what they want for their oral health
   B. Adolescents seek out dental care primarily to gain approval from their parents
   C. Adolescents respond to the same kinds of rewards that children do
   D. Adolescents do not need to be asked about their motivations for caring for their teeth

Exam Questions for Chapter 13:

Working With Orthodontic Patients

1. You are speaking with a 15-year-old male patient who is scheduled for orthodontic treatment. He tells you, "This whole braces deal wasn't my idea. My Mom's forcing me to do this." What can you assume from this statement?
   A. The patient will eventually "come around" and appreciate his orthodontic treatment
   B. You should keep instruction for home care limited at first
   C. He and his mother have a very conflicted relationship
   D. His orthodontic treatment is doomed to fail

2. What is a common barrier to working with adolescent orthodontic patients?
   A. They may feel forced into receiving treatment that they are not sure they want
   B. They do not have the skills necessary to keep their teeth clean with braces
   C. Their school schedules often get in the way of keeping appointments
   D. They are often careless with their orthodontic appliances
3. What is the rationale behind a "run-in"?
   A. To confront an adolescent with the consequences of poor home care
   B. To encourage parents to take an active part in their adolescent's oral health
   C. To improve self-care before placing orthodontic appliances
   D. To practice placing the orthodontic brackets on the adolescent's teeth
4. What is most important to remember to do when treating an adolescent after orthodontic appliances are placed?
   A. Rapidly introduce new cleaning tools so the adolescent doesn't get bored
   B. Keep your instructions simple and easy to understand
   C. Provide the adolescent with as many cleaning tools as you think she might need
   D. Assume that the adolescent will talk with her friends about the right way to keep her teeth clean
5. Which of the following is a symptom of depression that may be seen in adolescents?
   A. An adolescent who was doing well in school is now having academic problems
   B. An adolescent is now disinterested in an activity or sport that was once important
   C. An adolescent is visibly anxious or loudly argumentative and angry
   D. All of the above

Exam Questions for Chapter 14:

Adaptive Strategies for Patients with Special Needs and the Elderly

1. When should oral hygiene begin for a child with special needs?
   A. As soon as the first tooth erupts
   B. About 6 months after oral hygiene would be started for a child without special needs
   C. About 6 months before oral hygiene would be started for a child without special needs
   D. As soon as the first 6 teeth have erupted

2. Which of the following is NOT included in the "Lift the Lip" technique of examining a child's teeth?
   A. The child is positioned on his back, lying on the laps of adults who are sitting knee to knee
   B. The parents use a dental mirror and explorer to examine the child's teeth
   C. The child's head is in the lap of the parent or dental provider
   D. The parents are taught how to recognize "white spots" on the child's teeth

3. Which of the following may be used to help a child with special needs clean his teeth effectively?
   A. High-fluoride toothpaste
   B. Toothbrush with a large handle
   C. Toothbrush with a timer
   D. All of the above

4. Which of the following is NOT true about oral health problems of the elderly?
   A. The elderly have the greatest oral health needs of any segment of the population
   B. Elderly patients are more likely than younger patients to believe that many preventable losses, illnesses, and pain are an unavoidable part of aging
   C. Elderly patients are more likely to seek dental treatment than any other segment of the population
   D. Many elderly patients do not seek regular treatment, even as dentures no longer fit properly

5. Which of the following is NOT true about treating elderly patients?
   A. Providers should always insist on giving instructions to an elderly patient's adult child or caretaker instead of the patient himself
   B. Providers should give plenty of reinforcement to elderly patients
   C. Providers should give verbal and written instructions to elderly patients
   D. Providers should assess for psychological difficulties in elderly patients, such as depression

Answer Key

Chapter 1: 1) A; 2) C; 3) B; 4) A; 5) D

Chapter 2: 1) D; 2) C; 3) B; 4) A; 5) C

Chapter 3: 1) B; 2) A; 3) C; 4) C; 5) D

Chapter 4: 1) D; 2) B; 3) B; 4) A; 5) D

Chapter 5: 1) C; 2) A; 3) B; 4) B; 5) C

Chapter 6: 1) B; 2) D; 3) C; 4) B; 5) A

Chapter 7: 1) A; 2) C; 3) A; 4) B; 5) D

Chapter 8: 1) C; 2) A; 3) B; 4) D; 5) C

Chapter 9: 1) C; 2) A; 3) C; 4) B; 5) D

Chapter 10: 1) C; 2) B; 3) A; 4) C; 5) D

Chapter 11: 1) A; 2) D; 3) B; 4) C; 5) B

Chapter 12: 1) B; 2) D; 3) A; 4) B; 5) A

Chapter 13: 1) B; 2) A; 3) C; 4) B; 5) D

Chapter 14: 1) A; 2) B; 3) D; 4) C; 5) A